Your Best Pregnancy

The Ultimate Guide to Easing the Aches, Pains, and Uncomfortable Side Effects During Each Stage of Your Pregnancy

Jill Hoefs, MPT
Denise Jagroo, DPT, MTC, WCS

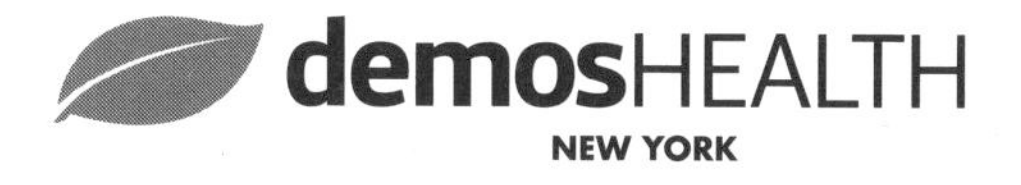

NEW YORK

Visit our website at www.demoshealth.com

ISBN: 978-1-936303-61-8
e-book ISBN: 978-1-61705-203-3

Acquisitions Editor: Julia Pastore
Compositor: diacriTech

Medical information provided by Demos Health, in the absence of a visit with a health care professional, must be considered as an educational service only. This book is not designed to replace a physician's independent judgment about the appropriateness or risks of a procedure or therapy for a given patient. Our purpose is to provide you with information that will help you make your own health care decisions.

The information and opinions provided here are believed to be accurate and sound, based on the best judgment available to the authors, editors, and publisher, but readers who fail to consult appropriate health authorities assume the risk of injuries. The publisher is not responsible for errors or omissions. The editors and publisher welcome any reader to report to the publisher any discrepancies or inaccuracies noticed.

Library of Congress Cataloging-in-Publication Data

Hoefs, Jill.
Your best pregnancy : the ultimate guide to easing the aches, pains, and uncomfortable side effects during each stage of your pregnancy / Jill Hoefs, MPT, and Denise Jagroo, DPT, MTC, WCS.
pages cm
Includes bibliographical references and index.
ISBN 978-1-936303-61-8—ISBN 978-1-61705-203-3 (e-Book)
1. Pregnancy—Popular works. 2. Exercise for pregnant women. I. Jagroo, Denise. II. Title.

RG525.H64 2014
618.2—dc23

2014027371

Special discounts on bulk quantities of Demos Health books are available to corporations, professional associations, pharmaceutical companies, health care organizations, and other qualifying groups. For details, please contact:

Special Sales Department
Demos Medical Publishing, LLC
11 West 42nd Street, 15th Floor
New York, NY 10036
Phone: 800-532-8663 or 212-683-0072
Fax: 212-941-7842
E-mail: specialsales@demosmedical.com

Printed in the United States of America by McNaughton & Gunn.
14 15 16 17 18 / 5 4 3 2 1

Your Best Pregnancy

To my three favorite people in the world: Mike, Aiden, and Zoe.
Jill Hoefs

To my family, for their love and support always.
Denise Jagroo

Contents

Introduction

We met in 2008 at a women's health continuing education class in Minneapolis. Upon realizing we were both physical therapists from Manhattan, we exchanged contact information and stayed connected. We frequently discussed our pregnant and postpartum patients. Some ladies couldn't sit while pregnant because of excruciating tailbone pain. Others couldn't be intimate because of painful scarring after their episiotomies. Many had low back pain that began while they were pregnant and never subsided. Some women were confined to bed and begged for exercises to maintain their strength for motherhood. Foot pain, rib pain, nonstop peeing, C-section complications.... The list went on and on. We've seen it all. Our postpartum patients would tell us about their difficult pregnancies and how many problems they encountered. They were told their symptoms were due to physiologic changes from their elevated pregnancy hormones. There wasn't anything they could do and their symptoms should resolve after their babies were born. They did not know that physical therapy was an option. Well it is! So for all our pregnant women struggling out there, you don't have to suffer. This book is for you. We understand everyone doesn't have access to a women's health physical therapist, so we brainstormed about how we could reach out to all women with problematic pregnancies. Our book idea was conceived in a Manhattan bar one evening in 2009 and there was no turning back. Over the next five years, we polled our pregnant and postpartum patients to determine their biggest complaints. And the list sure was long. We researched everything, spoke to countless experts, and then elaborated on their symptoms, treatments, and outcomes. Their stories are presented throughout the book to help you.

So please know, if you can't find a comfortable position, everything hurts, and you're waddling around town, you're not alone with your pregnancy complaints. That is why we wrote this book. We want to help you and have designed easy-to-follow exercises with clear instructions and photographs. To do the suggested exercises for different conditions, you will need a few supplies.

Resistance bands are a great strengthening tool, as you can easily increase or decrease the amount of resistance needed. Thicker bands offer more resistance and thinner bands offer less. They are color coded to distinguish the different levels of difficulty. Bands can be doubled up or used with more laxity to adjust the intensity. You can purchase them online or in a sporting goods store. (They are sold without latex if you have an allergy.) You can use light hand weights or household items such as small water bottles or larger plastic beverage containers. The resistance bands, water bottles, and weights are all interchangeable. Grab whichever is best for you. If you have room in your apartment or home, you may want to purchase an exercise ball. Please check the size chart to get the right ball for your height.

This book is designed to help you have your best pregnancy, even if you're off to a bad start. So read on!

CHAPTER 1

Ouch! What Is Happening to My Body? Help!

Ch-Ch-Ch-Changes…

How can two pregnant ladies look and feel so different? Some say they have never felt better. Their nails are strong and their hair is long. They feel beautiful and happy. They are trim and look like they're smuggling a basketball. They glow. And then, there are the not-so-lucky. They are tired, sore, cranky, bloated, nauseous, and hating every minute of their pregnancy. They can't sleep at night, but spend all day wishing they were in bed. They resent happy people. Their backs hurt. They feel like a sausage. And their boobs are killing them. Sound familiar?

From head to toe, your body undergoes a myriad of changes that may cause aches, pains, and discomfort. Read on for ways to treat these unwelcome symptoms and feel more comfortable throughout your pregnancy.

After talking to hundreds of patients, friends, colleagues, and doctors, we are ready to address the most painful pregnancy conditions. We understand we can't fix your morning sickness, preeclampsia, or raging hormones. But we can help you with back pain, pelvic floor issues, and discomfort stemming from your changing posture. So keep reading!

Red Flags

You may be experiencing one or more of the conditions mentioned in this chapter. If your symptoms, however, are very severe or if you are experiencing any of the conditions below, contact your health provider immediately:

Red flags during pregnancy include symptoms such as:

- Fainting
- Pain during urination
- Ongoing dizzy spells
- Vomiting and nausea symptoms that are extra persistent
- Sudden body swelling
- Rapid heartbeat
- Trouble walking
- Decreased fetal activity (i.e., far less than normal to no baby movement) for more than a day
- Sharp increase in fetal movement (could indicate fetus is in distress)
- Vaginal bleeding
- Early uterus cramping (such as weeks or months before your due date)
- Leaking amniotic fluid early on, which will feel a little like a constant trickling peeing sensation
- You have a general feeling that something is wrong—mamas have great instincts so trust your gut
- Severe abdominal or back pain (may indicate an ectopic pregnancy)
- Changes in vision (could be a sign of gestational diabetes or preeclampsia)
- Frequent, painful headaches (this may be due to nerve dysfunction, changes in hormones, increased blood circulation, preeclampsia, and other causes)
- All over itching late in pregnancy (if the itching is very intense, worse at night, and involves the soles of the feet and the palms of the hands, these symptoms may indicate a liver-based condition, such as obstetric cholestasis (OC))

Back Pain

Why do so many pregnant women have back pain? A lot happens in nine months! Some changes are obvious, some are not. The obvious change is in the size of your belly. Some women carry small, some women, not so much. Whatever the size, you will feel a change, as your core's muscular corset is offset. Your muscles and ligaments that once stabilized your spine are now being altered by the new tenant taking over your uterus. The bigger the baby grows, the less protection there is for your back as your abdominals stretch and your posture shifts forward. Your center of gravity is shifting forward with your growing breasts and abdomen and your muscles need to counteract to keep you upright. They work pretty hard in the end and you'll feel them! Keeping your core strong and stretching your muscles is important.

Lower Back Pain

Deb complained of low back pain when she was 25-weeks pregnant. She woke up during her sleep when she moved, often felt and heard popping with quick motions, had pain every evening, and was unable to hold her two-year-old daughter who forgot how to walk after learning about her new brother in utero. She complained of spasms on the right side of her low back and she often rolled on a tennis ball to relieve the pain.

What you can do

Strengthen your butt muscles

Your gluteus maximus should be the biggest and strongest skeletal muscle in your body. If it isn't doing its job, your smaller back muscles may get overtaxed as they compensate.

To safely strengthen your butt muscles, try the following exercise.

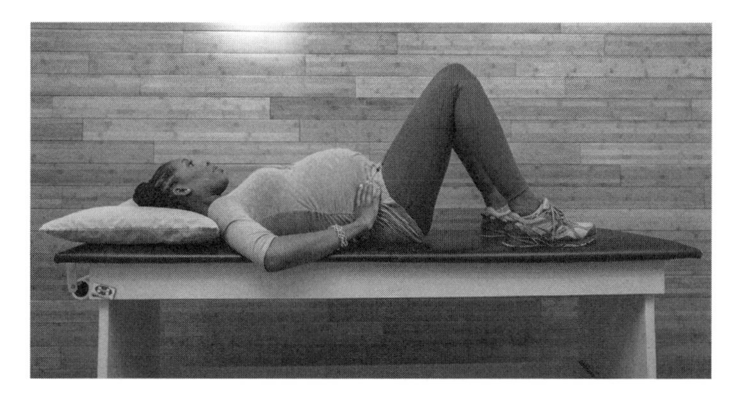

Bridges

- Bend both of your knees. Feet are flat and hip width apart.
- Tighten your butt.
- Lift your butt off your bed or floor.

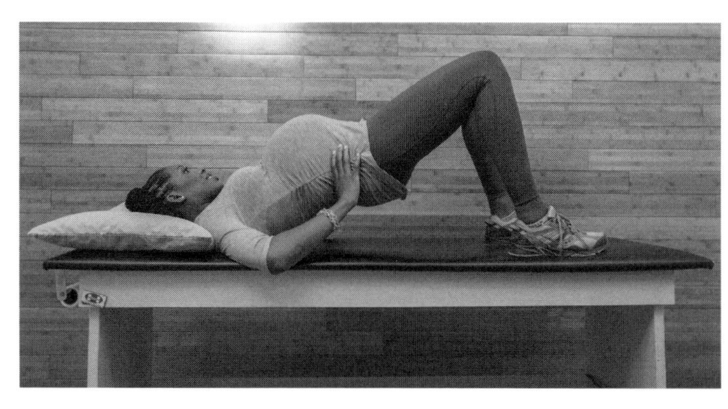

Bridging exercise

- Hold the position for three seconds.
- Slowly lower and repeat 15 times. Add a second set when this gets too easy.

Stretch your back and hip muscles

Tight muscles don't work efficiently. When they're not used properly, they get weak. When you eventually recruit them, they're deconditioned and painful to use. The snowball effect leaves you with tight, weak, and painful muscles. So here are some stretches to do to avoid this.

Core stretch (child's pose)

- Start off on your hands and knees. (We said earlier that it's not OK to be in this position. However, you're only spending a little bit of time in this position. You are moving quickly into the next pose where your belly will be supported on your thighs. So it's OK for now. And you are going to love this stretch so it's worth it to be on your hands and knees for a brief amount of time).
- Sit back onto your heels and then reach forward until you feel a stretch in your back.

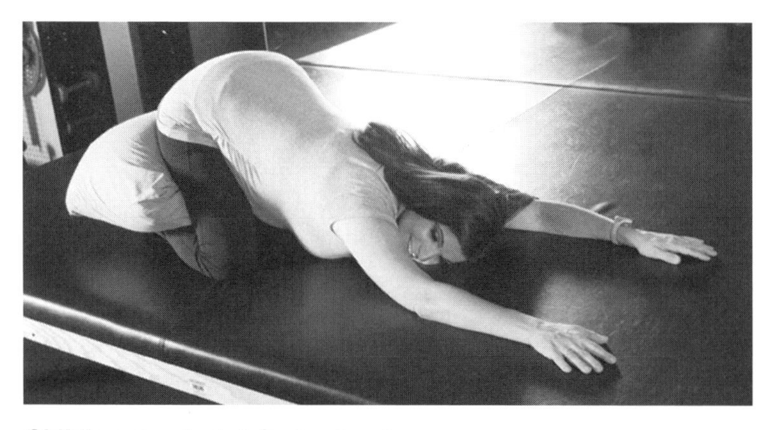

Child's pose stretch for back pain

You can modify this stretch by either separating your knees to allow a space for your belly and/or putting a pillow between your butt and ankles for comfort. You can also lean to either side to emphasize a painful side. For example, if your right side is more painful, reach your arms overhead to your left side while in the child's pose.

Hold this stretch for 30 seconds and repeat several times. Also, don't forget to breathe.

Rotation stretch

You can stretch your mid-back muscles and the muscles in between your ribs by rotating your trunk.

- Sit in a chair and sit up straight.
- Give yourself a hug.
- Keep your hips facing forward and turn your trunk toward the left. Hold that position for 30 seconds.
- Now turn your trunk to the right. Keep breathing and repeat.

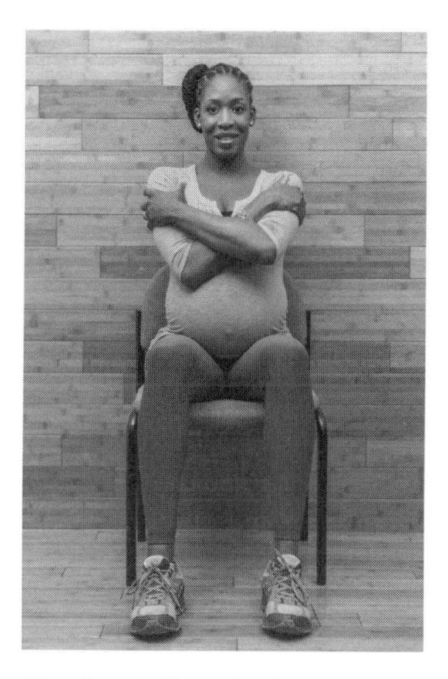
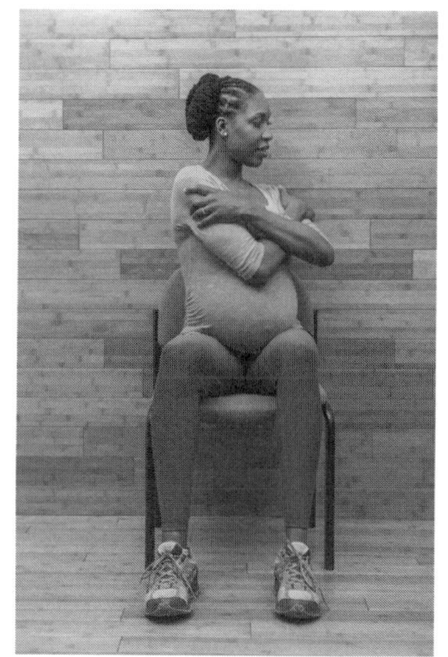
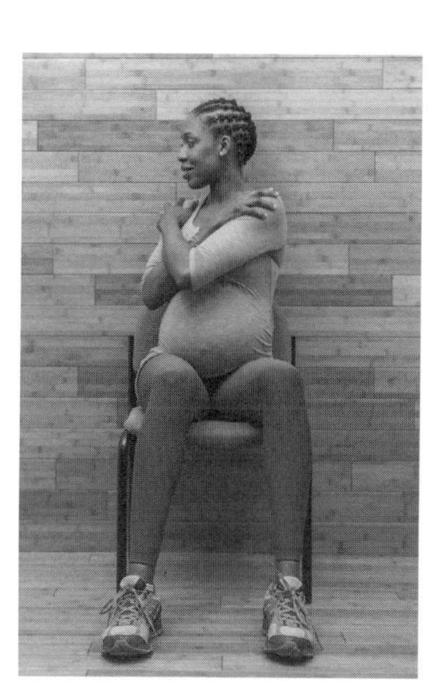

Trunk rotation stretch

Seated piriformis stretch

- Sit with your feet hip width apart.
- Rest your foot on your opposite thigh and lean forward, as much as your belly allows.
- You should feel this in your butt on the side of your crossed leg.
- Hold for 30 seconds.
- Stretch each side twice.

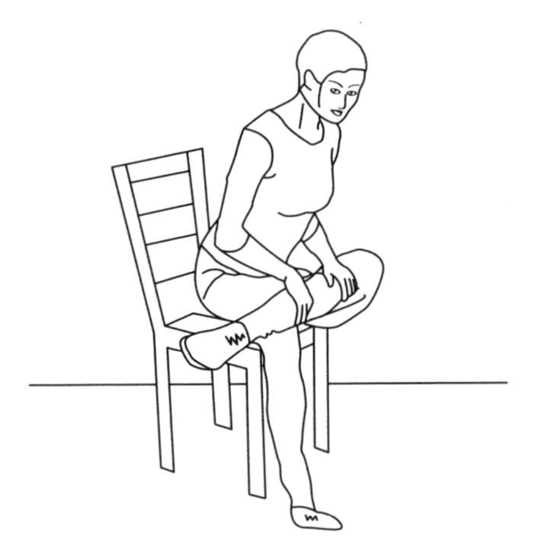

Seated piriformis (hip rotator) stretch

Some more tips for relieving/preventing your low back pain:

- **Avoid wearing high heels.** This will further shift your body weight forward. You need to wear comfortable and supportive shoes now.
- **Modify your sleeping position.** Refer to our section on sleeping pains (page 81). Steal more pillows if necessary, as you need to support your top leg while lying on your side. While changing positions, make sure to engage your abdominal muscles.
- **Engage your deep core muscles (your transverse abdominals) throughout the day**. Pull your belly button back toward your spine before lifting toddlers, groceries, laundry baskets, or free weights. Engage these muscles before getting in and out of bed, cars, or chairs. Don't shoot straight up out of bed. Instead, pull your belly button back to your spine and roll to your side before getting up. And lastly, engage these muscles before you cough, laugh, or sneeze. Your back will feel better when your core muscles are supporting it. For exercises to strengthen the transverse abdominals, see the section on separated abdominal muscles (diastasis recti) on page 63.
- **Walk correctly, no waddling.** The more efficiently you use your core muscles when walking, the less tight and sore you will feel.

  Refer to our section on correct gait mechanics on pages 34 to 35.
- **Use foam roller massage.** While it would be great to have a full-time massage therapist at your disposal, we know this isn't an option. Even our patients married to massage therapists have to beg for a session! Here is how you can massage the area on your own.

  Stand with a 6 inch × 36 inch foam roller vertically behind your spine. Lean against it and move your body side to side. This will massage the muscles adjacent to your spine. Do this for one minute.

  You can also turn the foam roller so that it is perpendicular to your spine and do some mini wall squats. As you squat down, the foam roller will move up your back and relieve tension in your back muscles. Good multitasking!

  Do 10 to 15 squats.

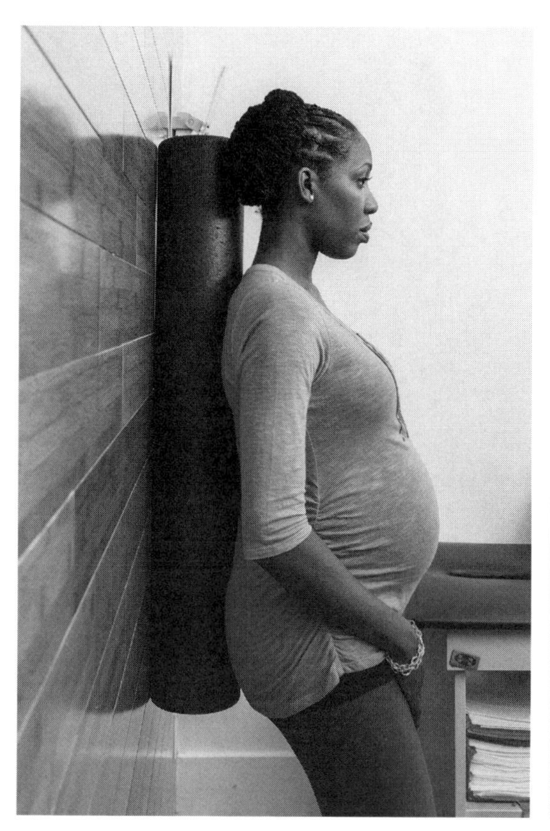
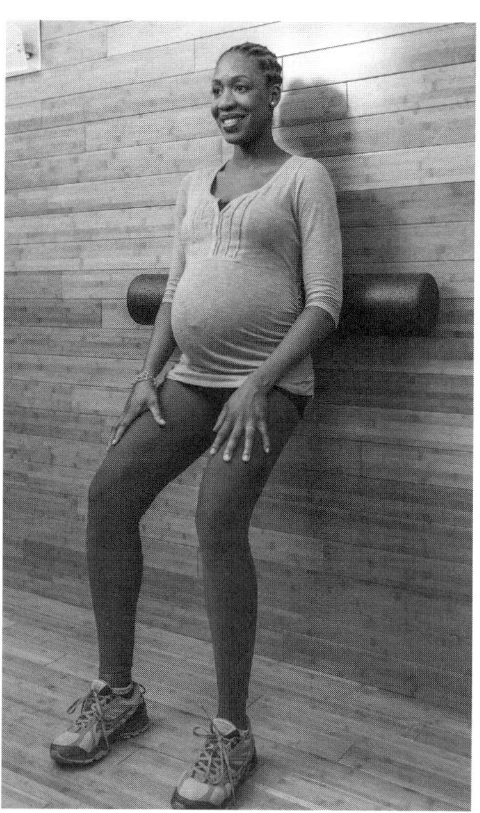

Foam rolling in standing for low back pain

Massage therapy

Doesn't a massage sound nice right about now? We consulted with licensed massage therapist Nicole Kruck, LMT, to share some special tips she uses when treating pregnant clients for low back pain. Grab your partner for this one. Nicole is certified in Women's Health and Reproductive Care, specializing in Fertility Enhancement, Prenatal & Postpartum Massage and Maya Abdominal Massage. "I have a great technique for low back pain or sacroiliac joint pain, both while pregnant and during labor. You can use a large sturdy scarf called a rebozo or a twin sheet. Fold the sheet or scarf so that it covers your hips (about 12 inches to 18 inches wide). Lie on your back and place the middle of the sheet just under your hips. Have your partner stand next to you, holding one end of the sheet in each hand. He or she will raise one side higher and then back down in a slow rocking motion. Allow three seconds with the sheet raised on one side before raising

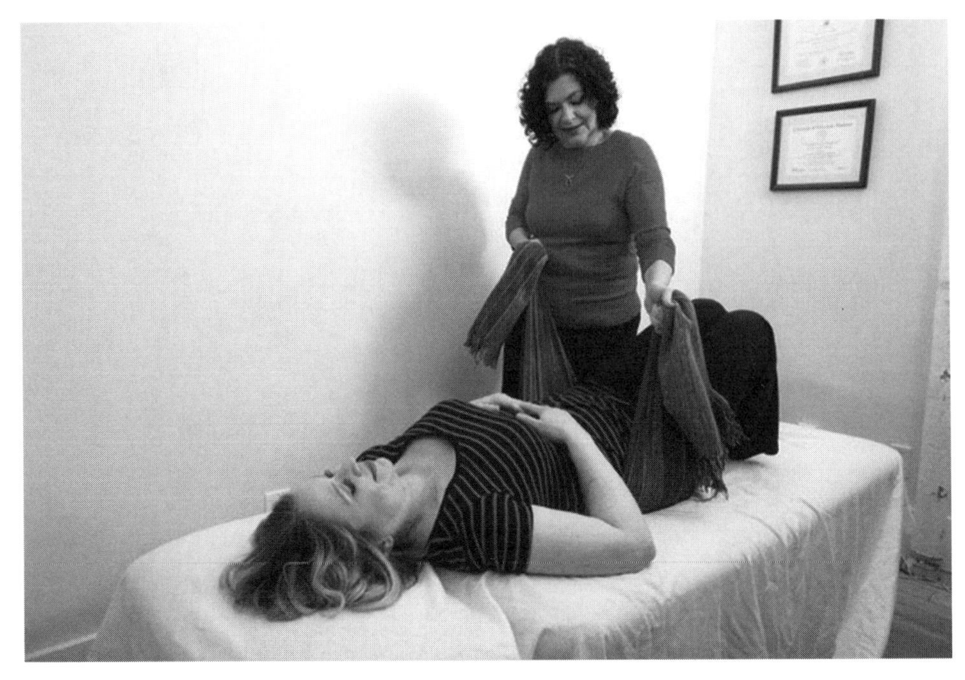

Using a rebozo for low back pain

Pregnant Employees, Rights in the Workplace

In 1978, Congress passed the Pregnancy Discrimination Act (PDA) to protect pregnant workers from discrimination in the workplace. That, along with the Americans with Disabilities Amendments Act (ADAAA), guarantees the right not to be treated adversely because of pregnancy, childbirth, or related medical conditions and requires employers to provide reasonable accommodation. A reasonable accommodation is a modification or adjustment that enables a person to do the core parts of his or her job. So what is a reasonable accommodation for pregnant employees? Modified work schedules, modified workplace policies (allowing a pregnant employee to drink water in a "no drinks allowed" area), reassignment to a vacant position, providing or modifying equipment (setting up an appropriate workstation), job restructuring, or light duty. So ladies, you don't have to tough it out if you're in pain. Modifications can be made. It's the law!

the other side for one to two minutes. This should bring relief for your low back pain and gently stretch the sacroiliac joints." Please do not try this if you are on bed rest or have placenta previa, as it is contraindicated.

Deb's back pain improved quickly. She modified her sleeping position to support her top leg while sleeping on her side. She said this helped her sleep for longer periods of time before needing to move. When she did change positions, she engaged her core muscles and moved slowly. Her favorite stretch was the child's pose. She did this stretch whenever she felt tight and it prevented her muscles from seizing up. She massaged her back muscles while standing against the foam roller, which she kept at her office. This lessened her pain most nights. Her daughter stopped asking to be carried. She relearned how to walk when she received new pink flashing sneakers as a big-sister-present. Phew!

In Case You Need Even More Reasons to Get a Massage

According to a recent study:

- Massage therapy has been demonstrated to be effective during pregnancy. The women reported decreased depression, anxiety, and leg and back pain.
- Depressed pregnant women given the pregnancy massage experienced fewer prenatal complications.
- The women who received massage therapy in the study experienced significantly less pain, and their labors were on average three hours shorter with less need for medication.
- There was a lower incidence of prematurity and low birthweight in the massaged depressed women.
- Postpartum depression and cortisol levels were decreased in the massaged women. The newborns of the massaged mothers also had lower cortisol levels than the newborns of the control mothers, and performed better on the Brazelton Neonatal Behavioral Assessment habituation, orientation, and motor scales.

Upper Back and Shoulder Pain

Olivia came to us for help with her upper back, shoulder, and neck pain. She hadn't gained much weight during her first trimester, but what she did gain was all in her chest and abdomen. She was buying new bras every three weeks and was worried she wouldn't be able to stand by the end of her pregnancy. Olivia was a dancer with amazing flexibility. While this enhanced her dance performance, it also contributed to some of her previous injuries, as she wasn't strong enough to stabilize her loose joints. Now that her pregnancy hormones were rising, she felt even more unstable and her muscles were working on overdrive to hold her together.

Her posture changed as her center of gravity shifted forward with her expanding belly and chest. She wasn't dancing as much, so her muscles weren't as strong as they used to be. Her once beautiful posture was now slumped forward and she needed some help. Her shoulder muscles ached and her upper back was killing her.

We know it is difficult to scold a woman to stand straight when her belly and breasts may be pulling her forward. But we'll do it anyway because we want to help you! Women often experience shoulder and upper back pain from engorged breasts, changes in posture, different sleep positions, and poor body mechanics during their pregnancy. (According to the March of Dimes, women can gain two pounds in their breasts alone!)

As your pregnancy progresses, there is more stress on your upper back muscles. Your center of gravity shifts forward and your muscles are working hard to maintain your posture. Feel the muscles between your breasts and your armpits. Are they sore? These muscles are your pectoralis minor muscles. If you're sitting or standing with hunched shoulders, they will tighten up. Ideally, your shoulders should be situated under your ears, not in front of them. But most things in life are in front of you—your desk, dinner table, baby(ies), steering wheel.... So it is common for these muscles to be tight and sore.

What you can do

Wear right size bra

It's important to wear the right size bra, as an incorrect fit can put too much pressure on the girls and can cause mastitis (inflammation of the mammary glands) and plugged milk ducts. Additionally, supportive bras will help prevent unnecessary strain on your neck and shoulders.

We know pregnancy comes with a lot of expenses. But skimping on good bras will contribute to upper body pain and discomfort. This pain will be worse than that on your wallet. While we recommend you visit a department store or lingerie shop to have a bra expert help you select the best bra, here are some tips if you're shopping solo.

A bra fits well if:

- It's not too tight or too loose.
- Your breasts fill the cup of the bra leaving no loose fabric and contain the whole breast without any bulging at the top, bottom, or sides.
- The strap at the back doesn't cut in.
- The shoulder straps don't carry the full weight of your breasts, stay in place when you lift your arms above your head, and fit closely to your body without digging in.
- The strap round the back and the front underband lie close to your body and are at the same level at the front and back.
- With an underwire bra, the underwire lies flat against your body and supports the underneath and sides of your breast without digging in or gaping.

It is sometimes suggested that pregnant women shouldn't wear underwire bras as the wiring can sometimes cause blockages in the milk ducts. However, there is no evidence to support this. As long as the bra fits you well and the wires of the bra aren't digging in, there is no reason to stop wearing an underwired bra.

However, you may find it more comfortable to wear a maternity or soft cup bra. These types of bras can also be worn in bed if you feel you need extra support while sleeping.

Support for the Boobs

Are your boobs driving you crazy yet? According to Jené Luciani in *The Bra Book*, 85 percent of women wear the wrong size bra. If this is true for the general public, imagine how ill-fitted the pregnant gals are! Their elevated estrogen and progesterone levels are visible in their newly acquired huge breasts. A woman's breasts can grow one to several cup sizes during pregnancy to prepare for lactation. For some women, this is a delight! Others complain that their breasts feel itchy from the stretched skin and extra sore from the increased volume. Breast growth traditionally begins at six to eight weeks and continues until 36 weeks, when it plateaus. But they're not done; they will grow another one to two sizes as your milk comes in.

Stretch your pectorals

You can open your chest and stretch your pectorals with the following exercise to decrease the tightness. These stretches can be performed in a doorway or corner.

- Place your forearms on each side of the doorway.
- Stand with your feet hip width apart.
- Lean forward through the open doorway while keeping your forearms flush against the wall. Feel the stretch in the front of your chest and shoulders.
- Hold for 30 seconds and repeat with your arms positioned higher and lower to target all your pectoral muscle fibers.

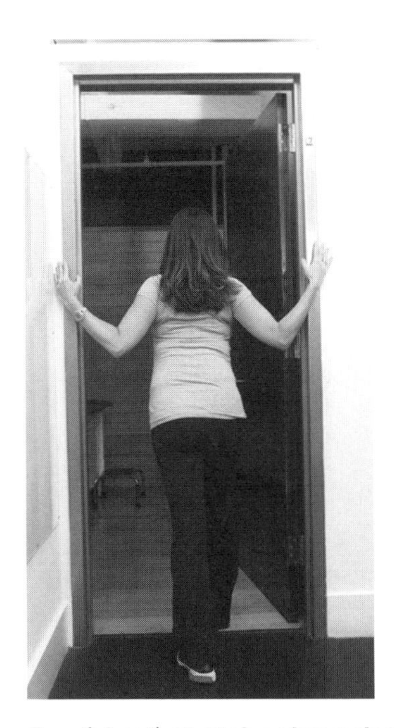
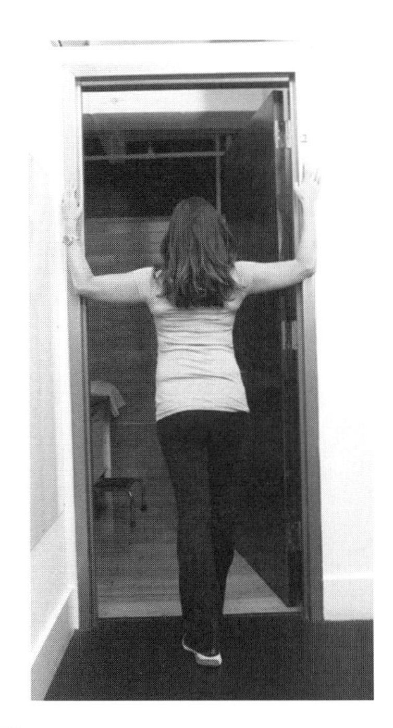
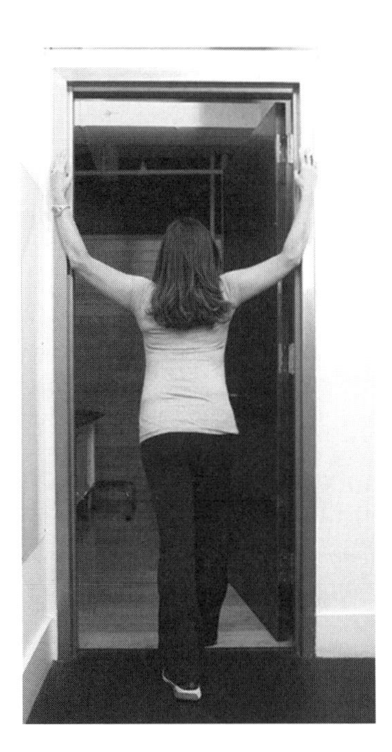

Pec (chest) stretch using a doorway

You can also perform "wall angels" to open your chest and work on your posture. This is just like making snow angels, but your legs are not involved. And there is no snow.

Stand with your back against a wall. (You can also do this sitting in a chair with your back against the wall.)

- Bring your arms out to the side with your elbows bent.
- Raise your arms upward so that your fingertips meet over your head.
- Feel the stretch in your chest and upper back. Repeat this motion 10 times. And remember, no cheating. Keep your back flat against the wall.

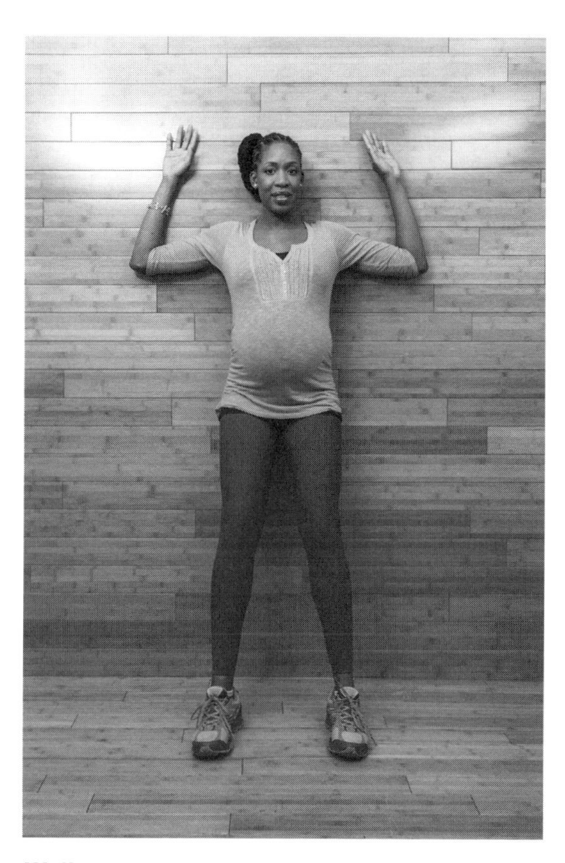

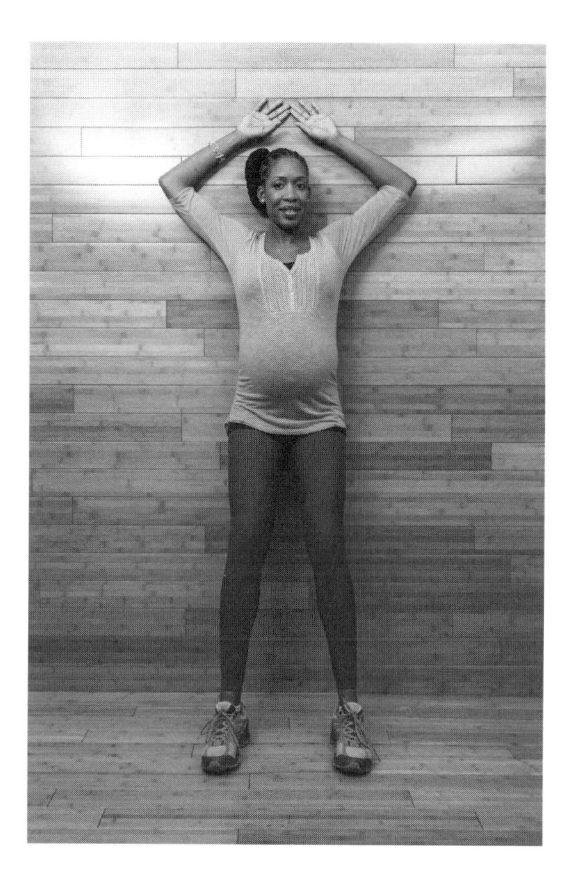

Wall angels

Stretch your upper trapezius muscles

You also need to stretch your upper trapezius muscles, the muscles that sit on top of your shoulders. Do you feel like you have the weight of the world on your shoulders? Well, you may, super mama. We don't doubt it. Or your muscles are just sore and tight and need some attention.

- Bring one arm behind your back and tilt your head to the opposite side.
- You can use the other arm to help gently guide your head forward, down, and to the side. Feel a stretch from your neck and all along the top of your shoulder. Hold for 30 seconds. Repeat two to three times.

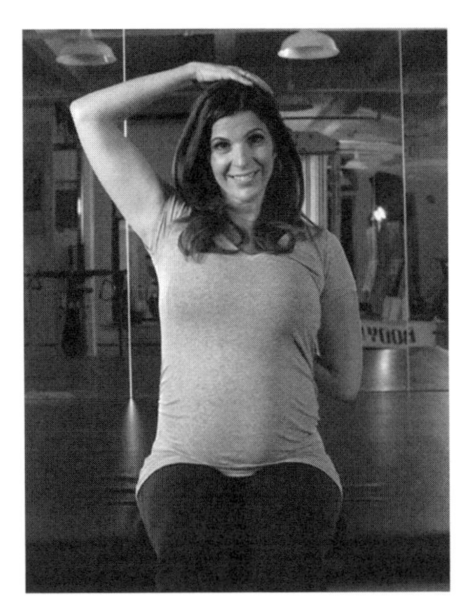

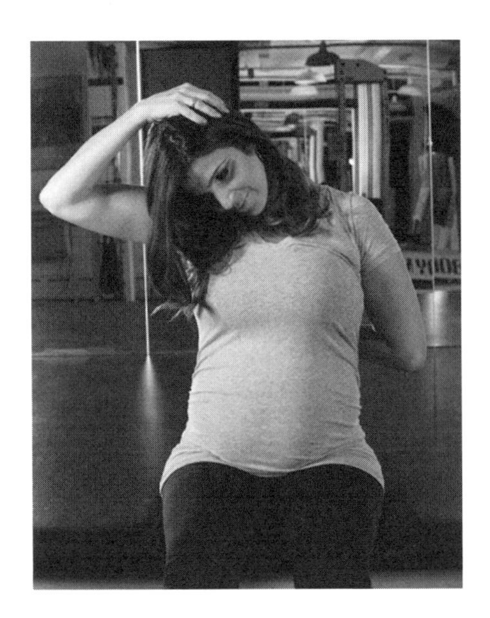

Trapezius (shoulder/neck) stretch

Stretch your neck

- Find a comfortable chair, sit down, and relax your shoulders.
- Tilt your head back, and look up to the ceiling.
- From this position, sidebend your neck, bringing your ear toward your shoulder.
- Feel for your collar bone on the opposite side. Pull gently down on your collar bone.

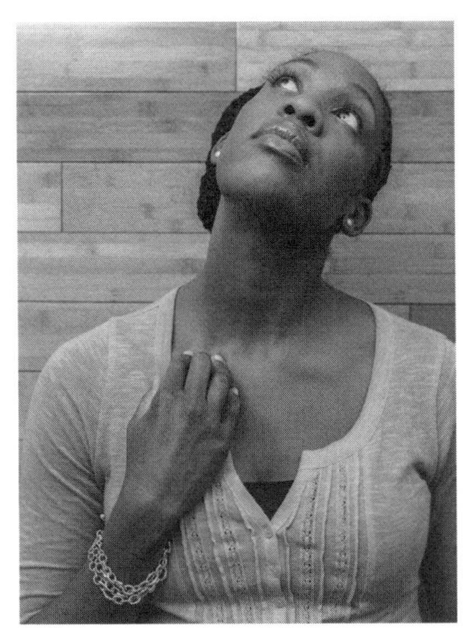

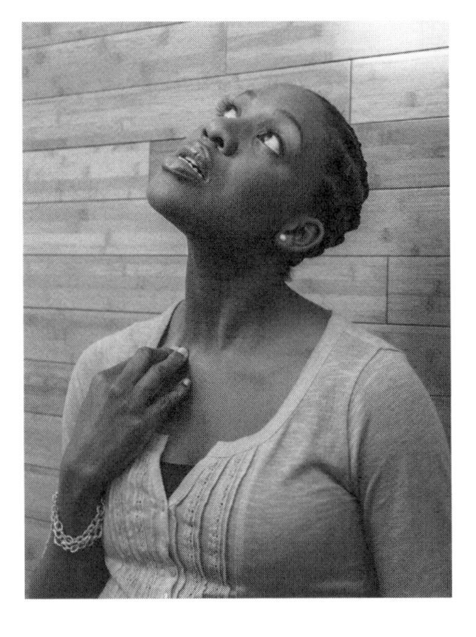

Neck stretch

- Stick your bottom teeth and jaw out.
- Feel the stretch in the muscles on the sides of your neck. Hold this position for 30 seconds.

** If you feel lightheaded in this position, please stop and notify your doctor or midwife.

Strengthen your upper back and shoulders

In addition to stretching your tight muscles, you need to strengthen the weak ones. As your shoulders round forward, your rhomboids and levator scapulae (both located between your shoulder blades and spine) are getting overstretched, and are thus inefficient.

- Grab a resistance band with moderate resistance.
- Hold the band with your palms up and elbows at your sides. Elbows are bent to 90 degrees.
- Squeeze your shoulder blades together while pulling your hands away from each other. Keep your elbows at your sides. Focus on using the muscles in between your shoulder blades to do the work, not just your arms. You can also perform this exercise with your elbows straight.
- Try two sets of 15 reps, every other day.

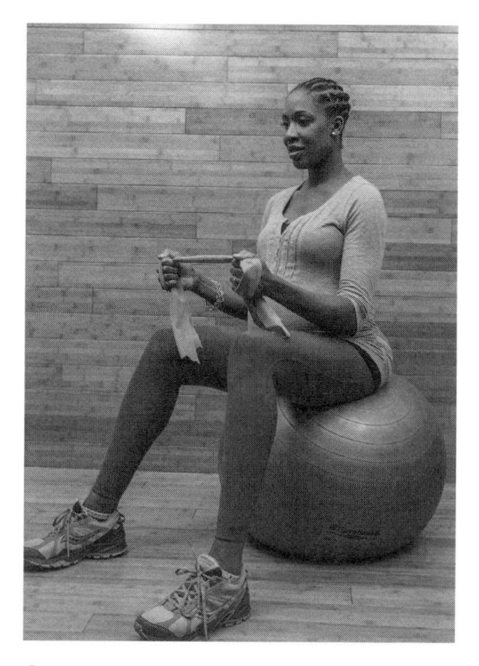

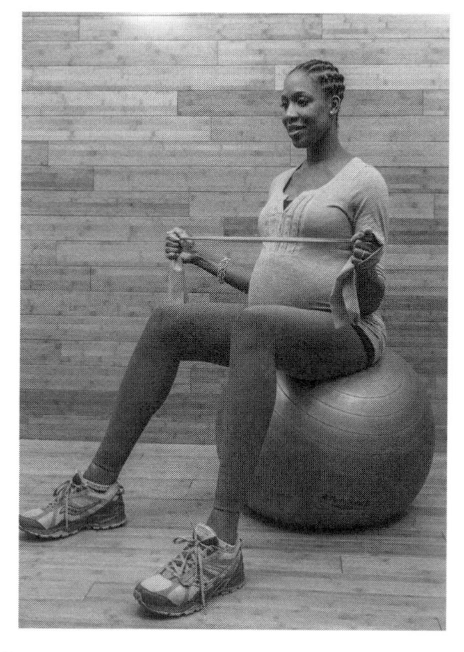

Shoulder blade squeezes, with elbows bent

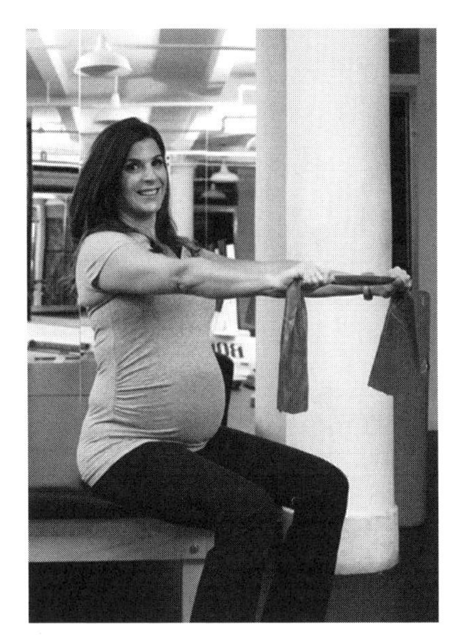

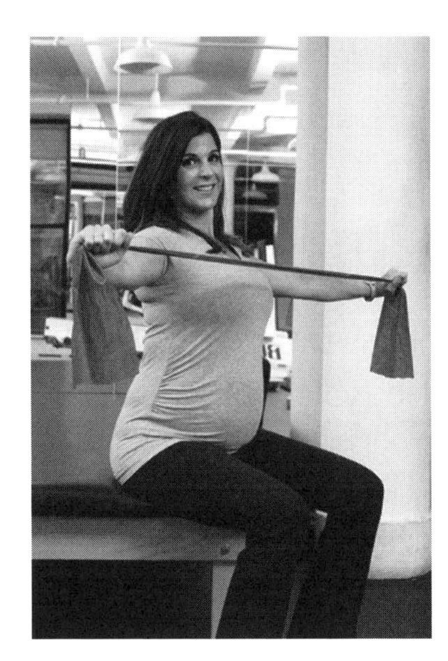

Shoulder blade squeezes, with elbows straight

Strengthen your pectoral muscles

Since you've stretched your chest muscles and have strengthened your upper back, try to balance the muscle forces by strengthening your pectoral muscles. Practice doing wall push-ups.

- Place your hands against a wall in front of you.
- Step about two feet away from the wall and keep your feet hip width apart.

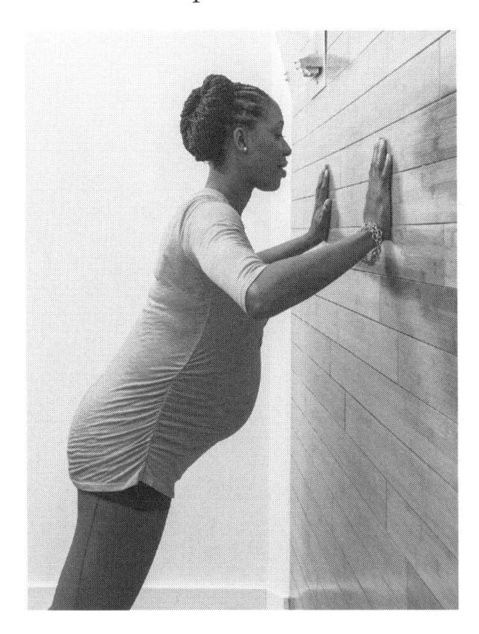

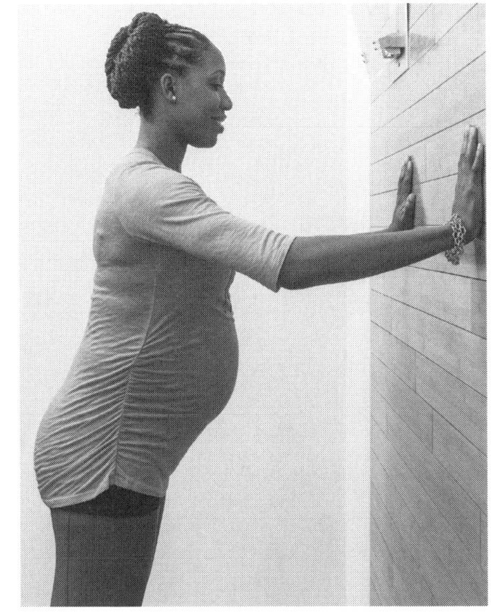

Wall push-up

- Keep your elbows facing slightly outward and lean your body into the wall. Make sure your body moves as one unit. Don't let your head or hips move first.
- Return to the starting position and repeat 10 times.

Use a foam roller

The foam roller is an excellent tool for stretching your pectorals and releasing tension in your upper back. It isn't quite as enjoyable as receiving a massage from a licensed massage therapist or your partner, but will help to decrease the tension in your muscles and bring healthy blood flow into the sore areas.

To stretch your pectoral muscles

- Lie on a 6 inch × 36 inch foam roller positioned under your head, spine, and butt.
- Bring your arms out to the side and bend your elbows so your hands and forearms can rest on the ground. This will support your vertebrae while allowing your chest and shoulder muscles to stretch with gravity.
- You can gently roll side to side to massage the muscles adjacent to your spine while stretching your pectorals. Get used to multitasking, as moms are great at this! Do this for one minute.

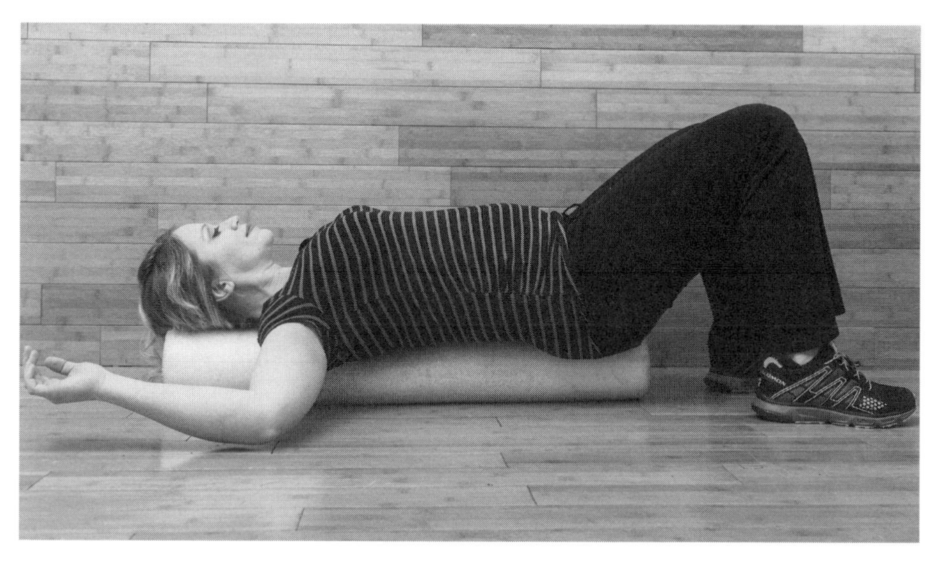

Using foam roller to stretch chest muscles

To release tension in your upper back

If the foam rolling isn't putting a dent in your tight muscles (pun intended), you might need to turn the foam roller perpendicular to your spine.

- Lie down carefully onto it and roll it under your upper back, wherever you are experiencing the most tension. You're now emphasizing a smaller area of your back so you're putting more pressure over it. This will feel like a deeper massage on the muscles. Do this for one minute.

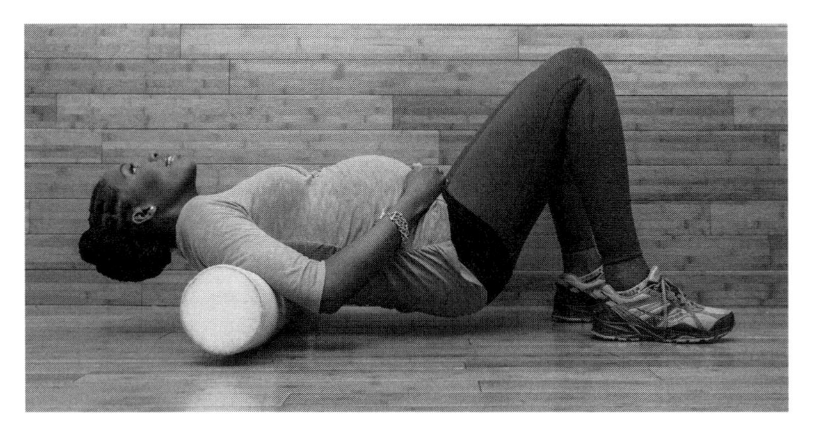

Using foam roller to roll tension out of back muscles

Mom Deserves a Massage

If your stubborn muscles aren't loosening with the foam roller, stretching, and corrected posture, it is probably time to locate a licensed physical therapist or prenatal massage therapist. If you are lucky enough to have a willing partner to massage you, make sure to conveniently leave this book open in a location where he or she can't miss it.

While lying on your stomach (or sitting if you are in a later stage of your pregnancy), your partner can massage your paraspinals, the muscles adjacent to your spine, with moderate pressure. He or she can use their palms or closed fists, whichever feels more comfortable, while emphasizing the tender areas.

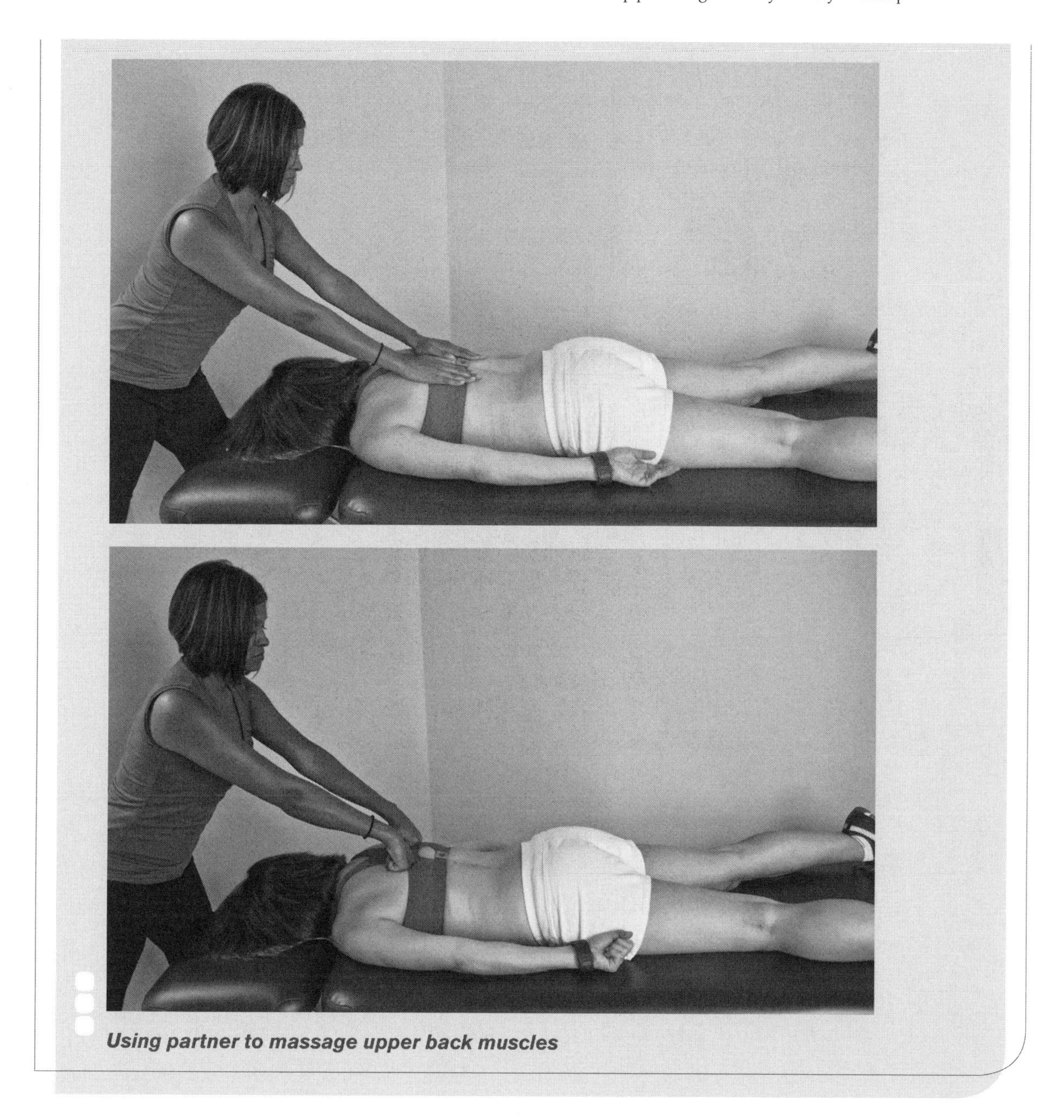

Using partner to massage upper back muscles

Stretching your chest and shoulders and strengthening your upper back shouldn't take longer than four to five minutes (whether in a doorway or on foam roller). Yes, you have time to do this. You will feel better.

Olivia loved having her shoulders taped back and down. Picture a soldier's posture. Now adjust so it doesn't seem as extreme. She would keep the tape on for two to three days and this reminded her how to stand, while letting her muscles

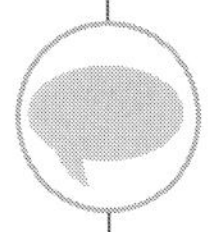

From Jill: I do a lot of taping with my patients. In this example, it supports your shoulders so your overworked muscles can relax. It is easier to maintain this healthy posture when you feel better and your muscles are less tight. You will be taught the correct stretching and strengthening exercises to maintain this corrected position. I would recommend finding a health care provider who has taken courses on kinesio-taping or McConnell taping. Both are great techniques.

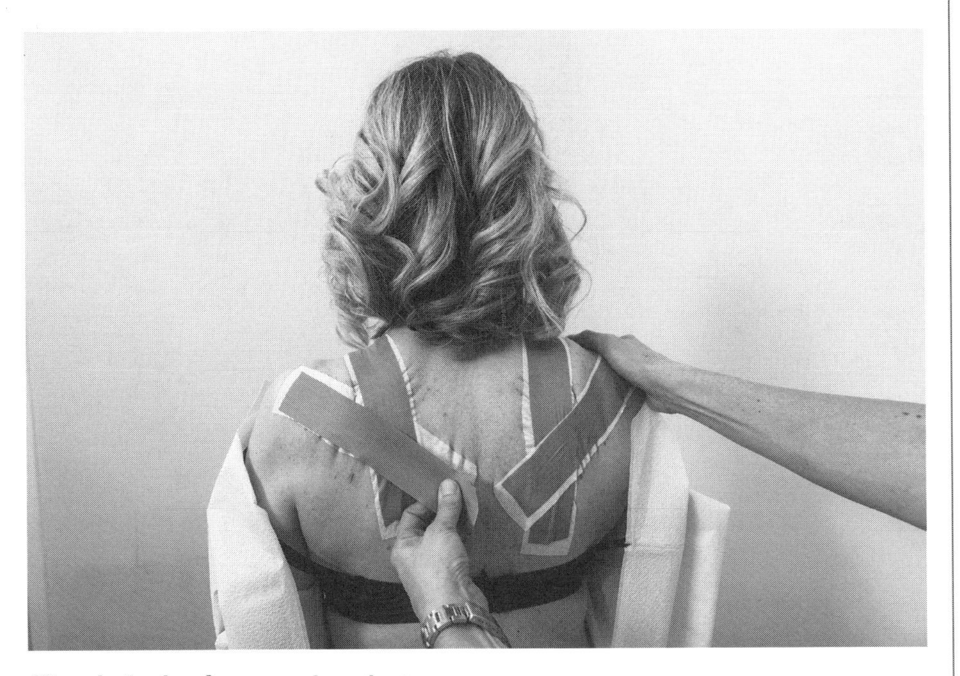

Kinesio-taping for correct posture

relax as the tape did its job. She did her strengthening and stretching exercises while the tape was on, and was able to hold her shoulders in the correct position when the tape was removed. Once she learned how to stabilize her shoulders, she only needed a couple sessions of physical therapy. She resumed her beautiful dancer's posture and her shoulder pain diminished. She was able to dance throughout her pregnancy (with the help of an extra supporting sports bra).

Bladder Issues

Cassandra's midwife referred her to a women's health physical therapist for urinary frequency. She was three weeks pregnant. We quickly understood the referral, as she needed the bathroom as soon as she arrived and again

50 minutes later. She found her incessant need to pee annoying, but was used to it, as it began four years earlier during her last pregnancy. She was afraid to drink too much water when she was away from her apartment for fear of not finding a bathroom when she needed one. She peed every one to two hours and three times during the night. She wasn't sure if she woke up because she had to pee or if she was just a light sleeper.

Does it seem like your bladder is the size of a thimble? You're not alone. We treat patients who complain about this day and night. Their increased frequency makes it difficult to work—especially when they need teacher coverage every hour to watch their classrooms. Our patients who get up three to four times each night to go to the bathroom are sleep-deprived and aggravated. All they want to do is sleep. We understand and want to help.

You shouldn't need the bathroom every hour while you're pregnant. You should only need the bathroom five to seven times a day to urinate. You should be able to hold your urine for at least two hours and up to five hours during the day. You shouldn't need the bathroom more than once a night and preferably, not at all.

Let's remember, the job of your bladder is to store urine and then empty it. Bladder and urological associations concur that a healthy bladder can accommodate one to two cups of urine, or three-quarters of a pint glass, before needing to be emptied. (Does that image help with your beer craving?) You can ignore that nagging bladder that wants to be emptied every time you sip your water. You can retrain the sensors in your bladder that are sending signals to your brain that the bladder needs to empty. You don't need to get up and go to the bathroom as soon as your bladder starts talking to you. Tell your bladder to wait. It will listen.

What you can do

Keep a diary

Some of you will remember an outfit you wore 10 years ago but can't remember what you had for breakfast yesterday. So you may need to keep a journal. This special journal is for your bladder. It will help you track how much you're drinking throughout your day, what you are drinking, how frequently you're skipping to the loo, whether you have urges to go, and if you leak urine throughout the day. With this information, you can modify your diet and voiding habits to improve your bladder function. The journal will show your improvement as you strengthen your pelvic floor muscles and retrain your bladder.

Sample Diary

DAY 1

	Fluids		**Urination**				**Accidents**		
	What kind?	How much?	How many times	How much? (s,m,l)	Strong urge to urinate?	What activity did this interrupt?	Did you have an accident?	How much? (s,m,l)	What were you doing at the time?
Sample	*Coffee*	*2 cups*	*1*	*M*	*Yes*	*Getting ready for work*	*Yes*	*M*	*Exercise*
6–9 a.m.									
9–12 noon									
12–3 p.m.									
3–6 p.m.									
6–9 p.m.									
9–12 mid									
12–3 a.m.									
3–6 a.m.									

Note the last time you went to the bathroom. Your goal is to wait at least two hours before going again. This may sound impossible. And for some of you, it will be. But you can do it. Think: Mind over Bladder. Start with small time increments (10 minutes, 20 minutes), then work your way up. Soon two hours will pass by and you won't even realize you held your urine the whole time. But don't show off. Once you get good at holding your urine, you don't have to hold it all day. You don't want to develop any urinary tract infections. Only camels need to store fluids for a long time.

There are many reasons pregnant ladies need to urinate frequently. Your blood volume increases, causing your kidneys to do more filtering and produce more urine. Your uterus may be pressing on your bladder. Your symptoms will improve during your second trimester, as your uterus grows and rises in your abdomen. Unfortunately, your baby will drop into your pelvis during your third trimester and the pressure returns. So what can you do besides wait?

Strengthen your pelvic floor

Strengthening your pelvic floor will help support your full bladder and uterus. This won't keep your growing baby from sitting on your bladder, unfortunately, but it can still decrease the urgency to pee. Try using Kegel exercises, which involve repeatedly contracting and relaxing the muscles that form part of the pelvic floor (see Chapter 3 for how to do these properly), to strengthen your pelvic floor. Reduce or eliminate the urge to urinate:

- Squeeze your pelvic floor muscles quickly several times when you get the urge feeling. To do this, tighten/squeeze and relax the pelvic muscle as rapidly as possible. Do not relax fully in between squeezes. Squeezing your pelvic floor muscles in this way sends a message to your nervous system and back to your bladder to stop contracting.
- As your bladder stops contracting and starts relaxing, the urge feeling subsides.
- Once the urge to urinate has subsided, you have a safe period when the bladder is calm. This "calm period" is the best time to go to the bathroom.

Just make sure not to practice your pelvic floor strengthening while urinating. Doing Kegel exercises while emptying your bladder can actually weaken the muscles, as well as lead to incomplete emptying of the bladder. This can increase the risk of a urinary tract infection, according to the Mayo Clinic.

Cassandra kept a bladder diary and, after two days, she was able to see that she was going to the bathroom more than necessary. She tried some of the strategies we taught her, such as waiting five to ten minutes before running to the bathroom and quick Kegels to retrain her bladder. She continued to use the bladder diary and saw some significant improvements by delaying her trips to the bathroom. Despite her growing belly and pressure on her bladder, she was able to wait two hours in between trips to the bathroom. She continued to wake up during the night, but that was just because she was uncomfortable. She would resist the urge to use the bathroom and fall back asleep.

After her daughter was born, she was too busy to keep a bladder diary, but she remembered our mantra: Mind over Bladder. She didn't go to the bathroom just because she was up to feed her baby or before she left the house. She remembered what we told her about New York City: There is a Starbucks on every corner and she will never be stranded without a bathroom.

Carpal Tunnel Syndrome

Caitlyn was a musician and lost sensation in her dominant hand while playing her violin. She had discomfort while practicing and picking up her violin case. Her pain and numbness were limiting her practice time and she had planned performances for another two months before her maternity leave began. Her company didn't offer disability leave. She needed relief so she could continue working and then care for her newborn without pain or numbness.

As if sleeping during your third trimester isn't uncomfortable enough. Now your hand burns, tingles, or gets numb while you're trying to sleep. And the not-so-lucky ones experience this in both hands. Carpal tunnel syndrome occurs when your median nerve, which controls sensation and strength in your hand, gets pressed and irritated in the carpal tunnel, located on the palm side of your wrist, near the base of your hand. The median nerve provides sensation to the palm side of your fingers, except for your pinky finger and outer half of your ring finger. It helps you move your thumb and fingers by controlling some small muscles in your hand. When there isn't enough room in the tunnel for it to move freely, the nerve gets pinched and your hand can feel numb and weak.

Why does this happen? It is three times more common in women, according to the National Institute for Neurological Disorders and

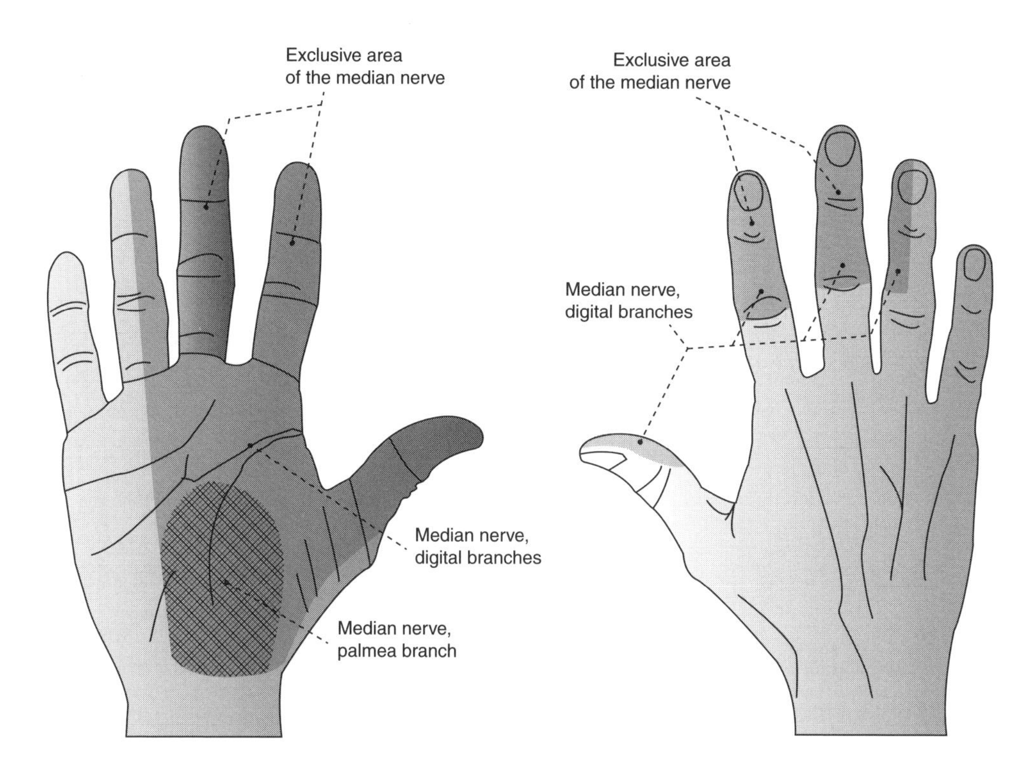

Strokes, due to their smaller carpal tunnel. This is consistent with a human cadaver study that measured the width and depth of the carpal tunnels in men and women. It was concluded that the shorter width of the tunnels in women may contribute to the higher incidence of carpal tunnel syndrome. It can happen during pregnancy when women retain more fluid, putting increased pressure on the nerve. Just like your legs swell during the day as you're standing, your arms and wrists can swell when you finally lie down. If you work on an assembly line and are pregnant with a genetic predisposition, then you're the unfortunate perfect candidate. You've got the trifecta.

How Do You Know If You Have Carpal Tunnel Syndrome?

There are two easy tests we do in our offices to test it. You can ask your partner to help you with these tests. And then earn his or her sympathy for having a pinched nerve in the wrist!

Tinel's sign test. With your palm facing up, have your partner tap the inside of your wrist with his/her index finger. If you feel numbness, pain, tingling, or pins and needles in your thumb, index, or middle finger, you might have carpal tunnel syndrome.

Phalen's sign test. Bring the back of your hands together with your wrists flexed and fingers facing down. Let your fingers dangle for about

60 seconds. If you feel numbness, pain, tingling, or pins and needles in your hand, you might have carpal tunnel syndrome.

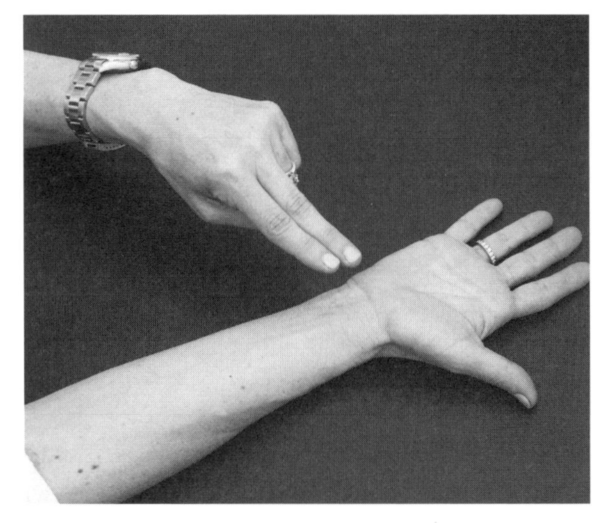

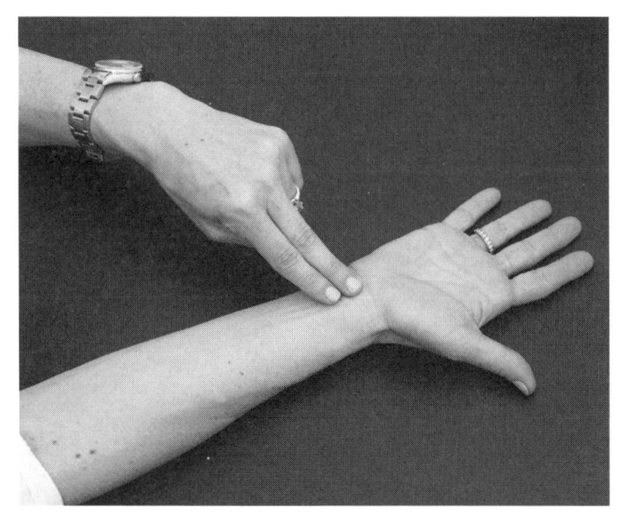

Tinel's sign test to detect carpal tunnel syndrome

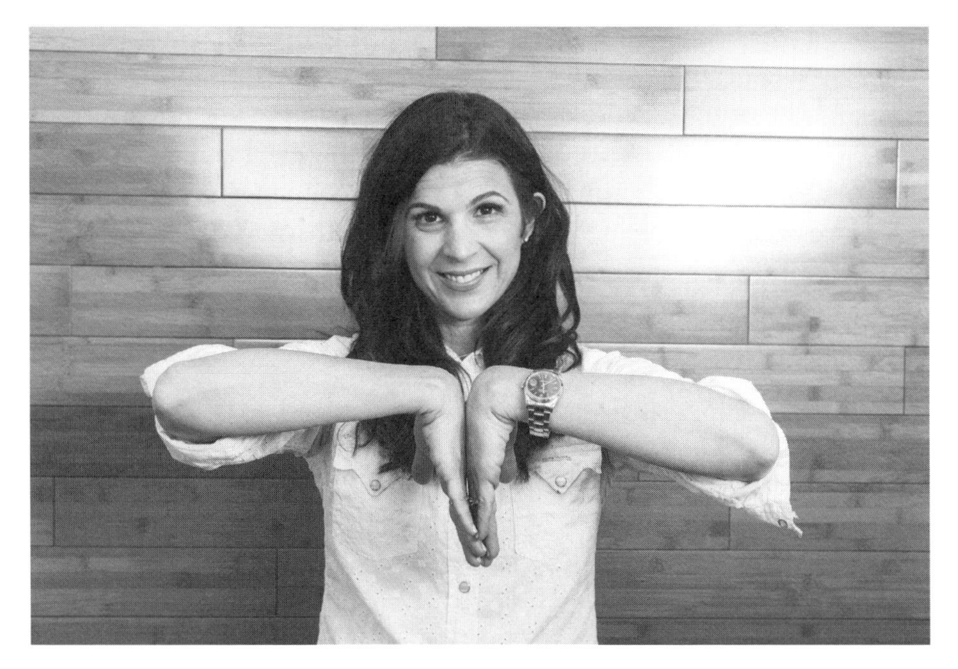

Phalen's sign test to detect carpal tunnel syndrome

What you can do

Some simple things you can do to mitigate symptoms include repositioning your arm, splinting your wrist, stretching, and exercising.

Pain-free and noninvasive treatments are likely to improve these unwanted symptoms during your pregnancy.

To minimize pressure on your carpal tunnel, you want to keep your wrist in a neutral position as much as possible. This means keeping it in line with your forearm and hand, not flexed or extended, as much as possible. Is your keyboard raised up in the back? If it is, then lower it so your wrists are in neutral and not extended. Your fingers and palms should not be lifted toward your forearm. This will only put additional strain on your wrists. Depending on your line of work, if this is not possible, at least try to keep it within a range of movement where you don't experience the pain. If you have a desk job, you should be sitting in a chair with sufficient support for your upper back and arms.

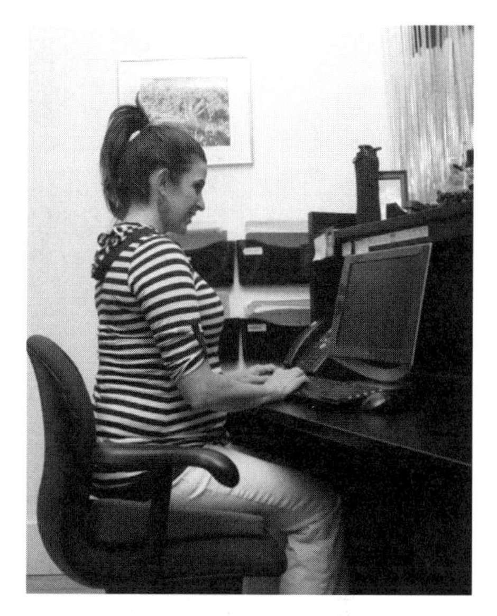

Maintaining proper wrist alignment at the workstation

Make sure to take frequent breaks throughout the day to relax your arms. You won't decrease your productivity by taking a one to two minute break every hour.

You can ensure your wrist will stay in place during your sleep by using a night splint. This is a removable device that usually attaches with Velcro and is semi-rigid. At the medical supply store (or online), look for a design that will keep your wrist straight without being too bulky and uncomfortable.

Stretch your wrists

- Straighten your arm and bend your wrist down.
- Use your other arm to apply a little extra pressure on the back side of your hand. You may feel a stretch up to your elbow. Hold this stretch for 30 seconds.

Another stretch you may want to try is called the "prayer stretch."

- Bring your hands together and position your palms in full contact with each other.
- Try bringing your elbows up and feel the stretch in the front of your wrists.

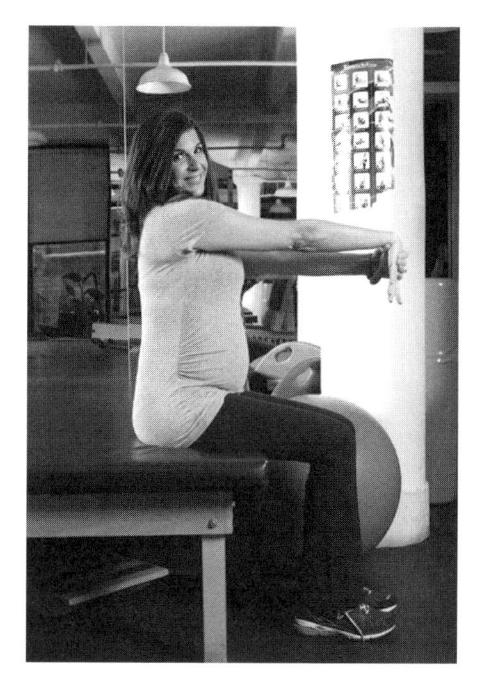

Wrist stretch

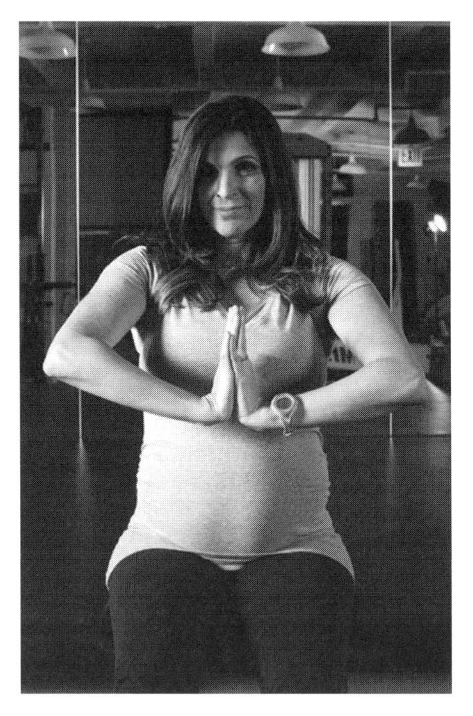

Wrist/forearm stretch

- Hold for 30 seconds. You may use this opportunity to actually pray for relief from carpal tunnel syndrome.

You can strengthen your fingers, hands, and wrists with putty, strengtheners (such as the Digi-Flex), or power hand webs. Musicians, athletes, and professionals who work with their hands frequently use these tools. They can be found in sporting goods stores or medical supply stores. They can be found online too, but we recommend you try the different levels to find the best intensity for you. You should be able to tolerate about one minute of strengthening two to three times per day.

To take the stress off your hands and wrist muscles, you can strengthen your large shoulder muscles. This will improve your posture and allow you to use your muscles more efficiently. Refer to the section on shoulder pain (p. 10) for exercises on how to strengthen your shoulder and upper back muscles.

If your pain is intense and these treatment options aren't helping, you may want to see your doctor and ask for a physical therapy referral. A physical therapist can apply manual trigger point therapy, lymphatic drainage, or soft tissue massage along the nerve pathway to alleviate tight points in muscles and soft tissue and move fluid that may be trapping the median nerve. Believe it or not, treating your neck and your upper ribs may help improve the pain in your wrists and hands. Additionally, a physical therapist can instruct you on nerve gliding, stretching, strengthening, and postural exercises to reduce your pain and improve your function. Based on your daily routine and work function, a physical therapist can also perform an ergonomic assessment of your home, office, or other workplace to ensure that you are positioned appropriately. Improving your posture and wrist alignment can relieve the stress on your wrists so you'll feel better.

Caitlyn purchased a night splint and wore it while she slept. This kept her wrist in neutral for seven hours. Before practicing, she performed the hand stretching and strengthening exercises we had shown her. Caitlyn was reluctant to begin an upper body strength training program for fear of injuring her hands. Once she did, however, she was able sit with better posture and not overtax her inflamed wrists. She used her shoulder muscles more efficiently to hold the violin, which allowed her to play with her wrists in neutral. Her carpal tunnel syndrome subsided after her pregnancy, but she continued her weight program. After all, her baby would soon weigh more than her instrument and she wanted to be ready.

Constipation

Gina understood it wasn't rational to be jealous of her two-year-old for pooping numerous times a day. Endlessly changing dirty diapers while pregnant, she wished she could poop half as much! Because she got so constipated, her biweekly poops were painful and labor-intensive. She couldn't possibly add more fiber to her diet, as she was already consuming high fiber cereals, beans, spinach, fiber gummies, and fiber bars daily.

So why do pregnant women get so constipated? Constipation during pregnancy occurs in 11 percent to 38 percent of women. The U.S. Department of Health and Human Services describes constipation as a condition in which a person poops fewer than three times a week and the poops are hard, dry, and small, making them painful or difficult to pass.

Blame it on the hormones once again. Your elevated progesterone hormone relaxes the smooth muscles in your organs. Smooth muscles found in your digestive system are different from skeletal muscles found on your legs. You can't voluntarily contract your intestinal muscles like you can flex your quadriceps. So you can't control your digestion. Your smooth muscles are found throughout your body in hollow organs such as the walls of your blood vessels and gastrointestinal tract. For example, these muscles control blood flow through your arteries, move food through your digestive system, and regulate airflow in the lungs.

When your intestinal smooth muscles relax, food moves more slowly, making bowel movements less frequent. With the delayed movement of food, there is more time for water to get absorbed. This results in stools that are hard and compact, making them difficult to pass. In the beginning of your pregnancy, you can blame your sluggish intestines and dehydrated poop for your constipation. Throw in the prenatal vitamins or iron supplements and it is even more brutal. Later in your pregnancy, your growing uterus intrudes on the territory that used to belong to your intestines and rectum. Your digestion system gets compressed, making it even more difficult for your stool to move along.

What you can do

What can you do since we've already said you can't control your intestinal activity?

- **Try to exercise every day.** Physical activity will help keep your digestive tract moving.
- **Increase your fiber intake** with raw fruits and vegetables, as much as you can. The Academy of Nutrition and Dietetics recommends consuming 20 to 35 grams of fiber a day for adults.

Examples of Foods That Have Fiber	Fiber Content
Beans, cereals, and breads	
½ cup of beans (navy, pinto, kidney, etc.), cooked	6.2–9.6 grams
½ cup of shredded wheat, ready-to-eat cereal	2.7–3.8 grams
⅓ cup of 100 percent bran, ready-to-eat cereal	9.1 grams
1 small oat bran muffin	3.0 grams
1 whole-wheat English muffin	4.4 grams
Fruits	
1 small apple, with skin	3.6 grams
1 medium pear, with skin	5.5 grams
½ cup of raspberries	4.0 grams
½ cup of stewed prunes	3.8 grams
Vegetables	
½ cup of winter squash, cooked	2.9 grams
1 medium sweet potato, baked in skin	3.8 grams
½ cup of green peas, cooked	3.5–4.4 grams
1 small potato, baked, with skin	3.0 grams
½ cup of mixed vegetables, cooked	4.0 grams
½ cup of broccoli, cooked	2.6–2.8 grams
½ cup of greens (spinach, collards, turnip greens), cooked	2.5–3.5 grams

Source: U.S. Department of Agriculture and U.S. Department of Health and Human Services, *Dietary Guidelines for Americans, 2010.*

- **Stay hydrated.** Pregnant women should drink as much as one eight-ounce glass of water or clear fluids (like herbal teas or broth) every hour.
- **Support your feet while on the toilet.** The squatting position helps your pelvic floor muscles relax. You can poop with less effort and strain if your knees are situated higher than your hips. We recommend a toilet stool such as the Squatty Potty to help you assume the squat.
- **Go to the bathroom when you need to.** Try to use the toilet at the same time daily and relax while you're sitting. Avoid sitting for too long, however, as this can make hemorrhoids worse.

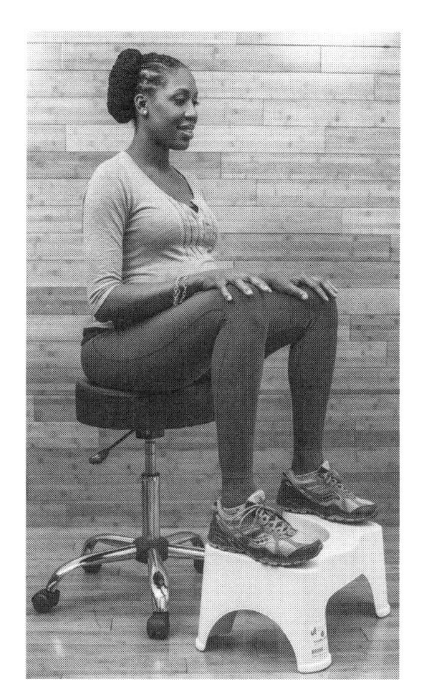

Squatty Potty

Tips for Treating Hemorrhoids

If you develop hemorrhoids, here are some treatment options that are safe for pregnancy and can reduce the burning or itching sensation.

- Take a warm sitz bath for 15 minutes as many times as needed throughout the day. Make sure to thoroughly dry your rectal area with a gentle towel.
- After you go to the bathroom, clean the anal area with a fragrance-free baby wipe or a cotton cloth soaked in warm water. Be thorough but gentle. Aggressive wiping can irritate the skin and make your hemorrhoids worse.
- If you feel sore, try this ice pack trick. Pour some water on a maxi pad, stick it in a resealable plastic bag, and freeze it. After a couple hours, stick it inside your underwear. Cover the top with some tissue or toilet paper so you don't freeze your butt off! This will help the inflammation and you will get some relief. Remove it after 10 minutes or less if it is too uncomfortable.
- Please discuss the use of topical creams with your doctor or midwife.
- Follow the instructions in the constipation section, as constipation contributes to hemorrhoids during pregnancy.

We approved of Gina's high fiber diet, but advised her to discuss her iron intake with her midwife. She was taking an iron supplement with 27 milligrams of iron daily, while consuming many foods high in iron. She was ingesting more iron than she needed. Her midwife made some dietary suggestions which helped her poop more. We suggested she use a Squatty Potty. Elevating her feet made it easier and quicker to poop. She found it awkward initially, but got used to it after a few days.

Heel and Bottom of Foot Pain (Plantar Fasciitis)

Kara came into the office and could only walk on the balls of her feet. She would wince when asked to put weight through her right heel. She didn't know how she injured herself, but she told us she gained 40 pounds in the past six months during her pregnancy. It was customary for her to take off her shoes upon entering her home but walking barefoot was too excruciating and she couldn't do it anymore.

Have you noticed your shoes have become too painful to wear? Don't give them away yet, as you may be able to wear them again once your baby is born. Is it because your feet are swollen? Maybe. Did your feet get flatter? Maybe. Is it because your walk has turned into a waddle? Maybe. As your center of gravity changes during your pregnancy, the way you walk and stand will change also. If you gain the expected 25 to 35 pounds, most of that weight is in your front, causing you to put more weight through the balls of your feet.

One common foot condition that plagues pregnant women is plantar fasciitis. Your plantar fascia is a thick band of tissue that runs under your foot. It starts at your heel and fans out toward your toes. It supports the arch of your foot and is integral in helping you walk.

There are many reasons it gets inflamed during pregnancy. If your extra pregnancy pounds are showing up in your thighs, you may walk with your feet wider apart to avoid inner thigh chafing. This will put increased pressure under your arches and cause inflammation to your plantar fascia. Changes in your feet can also contribute to the strain on the plantar fascia. According to the American College of Foot and Ankle Surgeons, women can experience a permanent growth in their feet, up to half a size, during their pregnancy. This was also seen during a 2013 study where women's arches were measured during their first trimester and again 19 weeks postpartum. Their arch heights and rigidity significantly decreased, while their foot lengths increased. It was concluded that pregnancy seems to be associated with a permanent loss of arch height, and the first pregnancy may be the most significant.

Your pregnancy hormones and pregnancy pounds can be blamed for your expanding foot. Just as your pregnancy hormones allow your pelvis to open for childbirth, they increase the laxity in your foot ligaments, making your feet spread in both length and width. When your foot expands in width, you will put more weight through the inside of your foot while walking or standing. This increased stress on your arch can inflame your plantar fascia, causing pain in your heel or under the arch. This is why you may hobble in the morning when you get out of bed.

How do you know if you have this condition you can't pronounce (PLAN-ter fash-ee-EYE-tus)? Many people have pain first thing in the morning upon getting out of bed.

- Are you walking on your toes because it is too painful to put your heels down?
- Is it painful to stand after sitting for extended periods?

What you can do

- **Stretch your calves and toes first thing in the morning**, before getting out of bed. (See pages 40-41 for calf stretches.)
- **Wear comfortable shoes and avoid flip flops.** Thin-soled shoes or flip flops should be avoided along with barefoot walking. The lack of arch support and cushioning of the heel while wearing flip flops or ballet flats can exacerbate your pain. You need to adequately support your expanding foot, so a trip to the shoe department may be warranted. So yes, you read this correctly: We're advising you to go shoe shopping!
- **Do this exercise to strengthen your outer hips.**
    - Stand tall with feet hip width apart and a medium resistance band tied around your ankles.
    - Take medium steps sideways while keeping your upper body centered over your feet. Don't let your trunk bend to the side. This exercise is to help you stop waddling … not enhance it!

You should feel your outer hip muscles work. If you bend your knees too much, this will turn into a quadriceps workout. You want your knees soft, not locked.

Depending on your space allowance, practice walking sideways in each direction for one minute. Some of our patients do this exercise in the hallway of their apartment buildings. Others need to change directions quickly as they try to find space in their tiny apartments. Work with the space you have and strengthen those outer hips

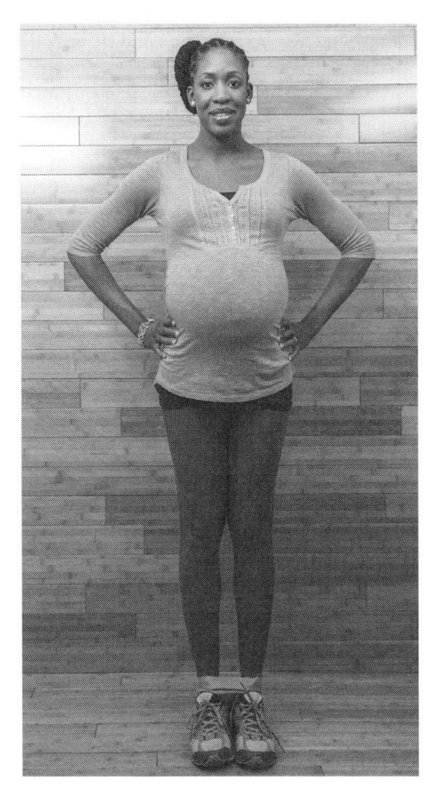

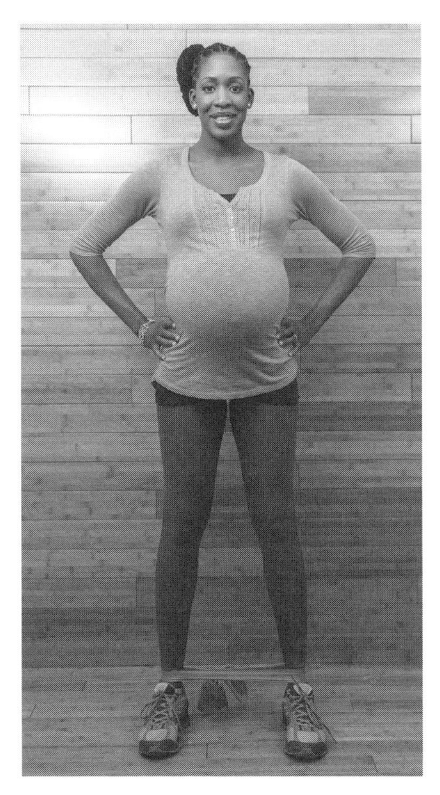

Walking sideways to strengthen outer hips

If this exercise gets too easy, you can double it around your ankles.

- **Try inserts in your shoes to lift your arches.** Generic inserts are fine during your pregnancy.
- **Ice the bottom of your foot** with a frozen water bottle first thing in the morning to decrease the inflammation.
- **Wear a night splint** to hold your foot in neutral so your plantar fascia doesn't tighten overnight. They aren't expensive and can be purchased in a medical pharmacy or online. However, many patients find them uncomfortable to sleep with. As if trying to sleep peacefully during your third trimester isn't challenging enough!
- **Work on your strut.** You don't need to waddle. We help women walk efficiently and with less pain every day in our offices. Here are some of our cues to walk with less discomfort.

- Take long and soft steps. The louder you pound your feet, the more your plantar fascia and bones need to absorb the impact. Lighter and softer steps allow your muscles to absorb the shocks better, which is what you want.
- Use your larger hip and upper body muscles. Let your bent arms swing and your upper body rotate slightly. You won't look silly and you'll be more efficient when you walk.
- Take longer steps more quickly. The more time you spend on your feet, the more they'll hurt. We want to avoid this. Taking quick steps is actually easier and less painful because you gain momentum to help you move.

The power walkers in Central Park have the right idea. They use their muscles so efficiently and have their walking technique down to a science. They barely spend any time on their feet. While we don't expect you to power walk to your bathroom in the morning, you will see the benefits of incorporating your upper body with this practice exercise:

- Walk with your straight arms glued to your sides and see how your feet feel.
- Then practice swinging your bent arms forward and back while letting your torso rotate freely. You should see this technique allows you to take longer steps more quickly, which is what you want. Now how do the feet feel?

If you have tried all the tips listed above and your pain is still limiting you from functioning at your full capacity, please talk to your doctor or midwife. He or she can hopefully refer you to a physical therapist. We will use different pregnancy-safe tools to help decrease your pain, such as cold laser therapy, tape, biofeedback (where sticker electrodes are placed on your muscles and connected to a computer screen to visibly see how your muscles are or are not working), and, best of all, our

From Denise: Swimming is a great full body workout that doesn't stress your joints. Just make sure you don't swim in a pool that is too warm. Remember that you are exercising and increasing your body temperature. Whenever I have aches and pains from triathlon training, jumping in the pool is a great fix. The buoyancy helps take the weight off your aching joints. Avoid kicking off of a pool wall if you have plantar fasciitis. It may increase the discomfort in your foot or cause a cramp.

hands. We will do a full evaluation of your posture, gait mechanics, strength, flexibility, and joint mobility and study your painful areas. We will determine what is contributing to your painful feet and teach you what you can do to improve your pain.

Flipflopitis

What is wrong with wearing flip flops? Nothing of course, if you're just wearing them in public showers or to the beach. However, after wearing supportive shoes all winter, flip flops are a shock to the system when worn for several hours a day. As you walk, you take shorter strides and curl your toes so your shoes don't flip off your feet and cause you to flop. This change in your walk pattern will strain your feet, not to mention your legs, hips, and back. Podiatrists get busy in the summer treating heel pain, ankle sprains, Achilles tendonitis, and other injuries associated with flip flop wearing.

Kara's feet needed some help. Luckily, she responded quickly to our suggestions and treatment. After observing her walk on the treadmill, we gave her some suggestions to improve her efficiency. She needed to use her upper body and arms more when she walked, and take faster, longer steps. This would take the stress off her feet. We also advised her to purchase wider and more supportive shoes. She objected until we traced her bare foot on paper and cut it out. When she saw it was wider than the sole of her shoe, she agreed to purchase new shoes. She began stretching her calves regularly and got weekly foot massages at her local nail salon.

As for walking barefoot in her home, she opted for a pair of slippers and was OK with this resolution.

Lightheadedness

Mia was struggling during her pregnancy with lightheadedness. She often woke up in the middle of the night to use the bathroom and, if she got up too quickly, had to steady herself by holding onto the walls until the room stopped spinning. Other times she would squat to the ground and wait until the dizziness passed, so she wouldn't fall over.

In your second and third trimesters, your growing uterus can slow the circulation in your legs by compressing the inferior vena cava (the large vein that returns blood from the lower half of the body to the heart) and the pelvic veins.

Lying flat on your back can make this problem worse. In fact, about 8 percent of pregnant women in their second and third trimesters develop a condition called supine hypotensive syndrome: When they lie on their back, their heart rate increases, their blood pressure drops, and they feel anxious, lightheaded, and nauseated until they shift their position.

What you can do

To avoid this problem, lie on your side instead of flat on your back. Either side is better than your back, although the left side is best. A pillow placed behind you or under your hip can help you stay on your side—or at least tilted enough to keep your uterus from compressing the vena cava.

Upon questioning Mia about her sleep patterns, it was determined that she was a back sleeper. Once she started sleeping on her side with a body pillow, her lightheadedness improved and she no longer needed the walls to hold her up. Now if only her bladder would let her sleep through the night!

Preg Head

Do you have Momnesia? Did you forget where you put your keys? Are you wondering if you already made lunch for tomorrow? Your raging pregnancy hormones and changing priorities may explain this. "There is 15 to 40 times more progesterone and estrogen marinating the brain during pregnancy," Louann Brizendine, MD, director of the Women's Mood and Hormone Clinic at the University of California, San Francisco, says. "And these hormones affect all kinds of neurons in the brain. By the time the woman delivers, there are huge surges of oxytocin that cause the uterus to contract and the body to produce milk—and they also affect the brain circuits. The brain also *shrinks* during pregnancy—it does not lose cells but changes metabolism and restructures. Then in the final one to two weeks, the brain begins to increase in size again and construct maternal circuits. It does not return to its former size until about six months after giving birth. You only have so many shelves in your brain, so the top three are filled with baby stuff." Hormones may also affect spatial memory—which includes remembering where things are—in pregnant women and new moms, a British study shows. It may be evolutionary as well. Not thinking or remembering other things helps you to put all your focus on caring for your newborn.

You can leave notes for yourself on the fridge or set reminder alerts on your phone to remember where you put things. You'll just have to remember where you put your phone.

Lower Abdominal/Groin Pain (Round Ligament Pain)

Dana was an avid cyclist and didn't want to give up riding when she found out she was pregnant. When her belly got too big for her to keep her balance on her road bike, she switched to indoor spin classes. Dana could barely make it through a class without having terrible pain in her groin on the right side and low abdomen. She had a tough time walking the next day, but couldn't find another form of exercise she enjoyed.

Your round ligament is often to blame for the abdominal pain during your second trimester. The pain can be achy as it stretches and thickens to support your growing uterus, or sharp if you move too quickly. It connects the front of your uterus to your groin on both sides. Your body is directing extra blood flow to your uterus, nourishing the area with oxygen and nutrients. This will speed up the healing. While this is happening, the baby is growing, moving, and turning … hopefully away from the painful area!

What you can do

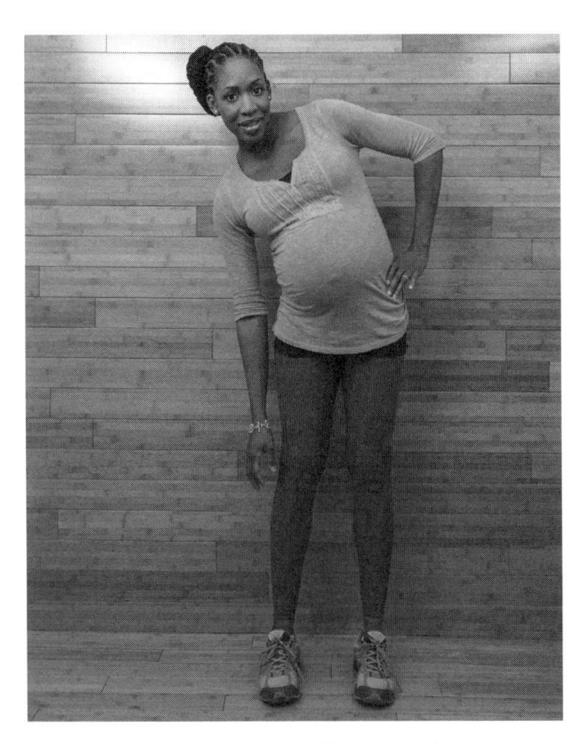

Round ligament side-bending stretch

- Avoid sudden movements from sitting to standing.
- Arise slowly from bed in the morning.
- Support the uterus with a pillow under the abdomen and between the knees when side lying.
- Wear an abdominal support garment.
- Stretch the round ligament by sidebending your trunk. Stand and lean in toward the side that hurts. This will put the ligament on slack and relieve some of your symptoms.

You can also try hiking your hip up while you are standing (the painful side). This will also slacken the ligament and relieve the strain on it.

Dana was able to continue her love of cycling … with a few minor adjustments. She didn't move into different positions on the bike when the instructor suggested. She remained in the saddle (on the bike seat) throughout the entire class. She only turned up the resistance if she felt she could tolerate it. She wore a maternity abdominal support garment throughout the day and sometimes during spin class. She only put her foot in the pedal "cages" if she felt her groin could take the resistance. She loved that she was able to still ride, even if it was indoors.

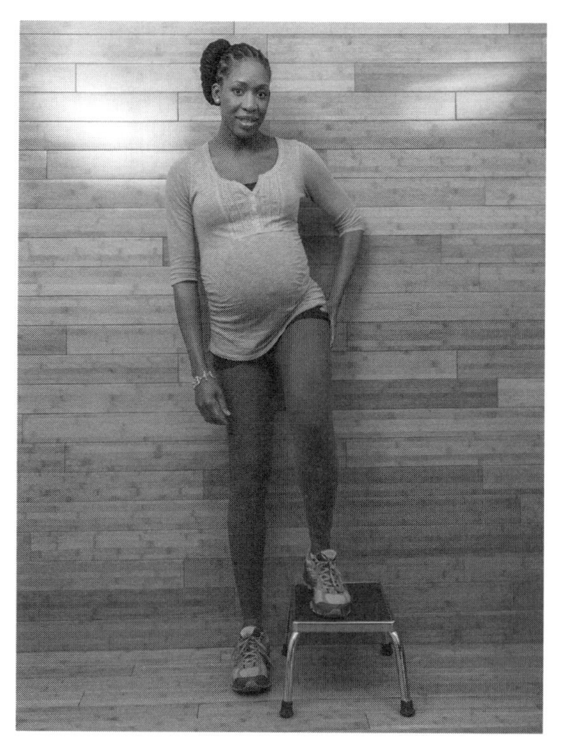

Hip hiking round ligament stretch

Night Cramps

Jessica was seven months pregnant and reported that she couldn't sleep longer than two and a half consecutive hours before she was awakened by sharp calf cramps in either leg. She described the pain as feeling like she was being stabbed in the calf by an ice pick. She moved back and forth between the couch and her bed, as she felt bad about keeping her husband awake too. She dreaded going to bed, as she knew she would awaken with pain and be irritable in the morning from lack of sleep. She was struggling at work, was too tired to exercise, and couldn't wait for her pregnancy to end. She modified her diet to include more bananas and potassium, but still couldn't sleep through the night.

We hope you never experience this, but if you're one of the unlucky ones that has, you know how painful these calf cramps can be. Studies show that during pregnancy, up to 30 percent of women can be affected by leg cramps. Why do they occur? One reason is that the growing uterus increases the pressure in the pelvis, reducing blood flow to the legs. Cramping is the triplet sister to swelling and varicose veins. Cramps feel like charley horses and can happen during the second half of your pregnancy, frequently or intermittently.

After discussing calf cramp prevention with numerous doctors and combing the literature, we have many helpful suggestions, but no cures. Sorry! Even though a definite cure doesn't exist, our

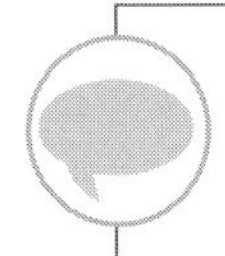

From Jill: While pregnant I learned that saying a quick wish before going to bed didn't help. Even though the spasms only lasted a few seconds, my potty mouth was active the second they began. Conversations with my husband sounded like this:

"Oh f@%k, not again! *Quick, help me stretch it."*

"Like this?"

"No, that kills. Try massaging it. But not that hard!!!"

"OK, just relax."

" I can't relax! My leg is f-ing killing me. I need to walk."

"I will help you."

"Never mind, its subsiding. Thank you. Good night."

patients, doctors, and colleagues shared their remedies. These recommendations have helped many patients and we hope they will help you too.

What you can do

- Move your feet in circles to improve circulation—both clockwise and counterclockwise throughout the day.
- Stretch your calves.
- Stay hydrated.
- Be extra nice to your partner so he or she will give you a calf massage.

How can you stretch your calves? The calves can be stretched without any devices or by using a stretching tool such as the ProStretch. You will want to stretch your outer gastrocnemius muscle with your knee straight and the underlying soleus muscle with your knee bent.

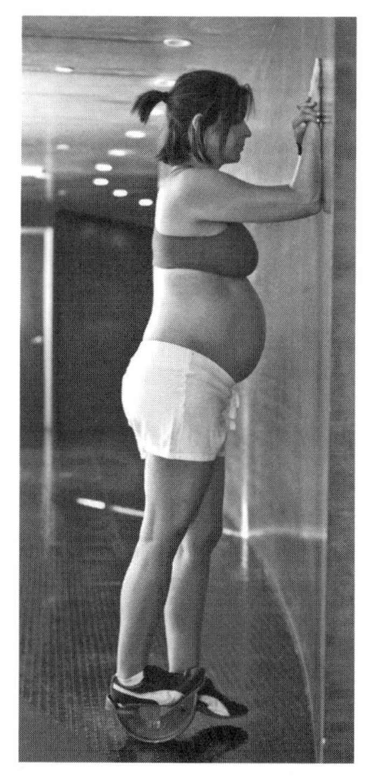

Calf stretch with the proStretch device

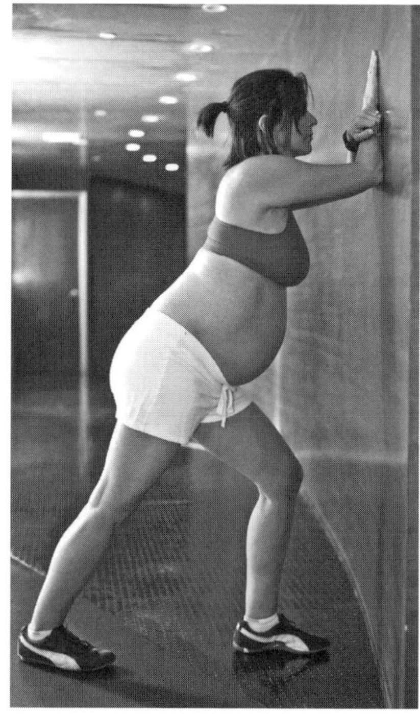

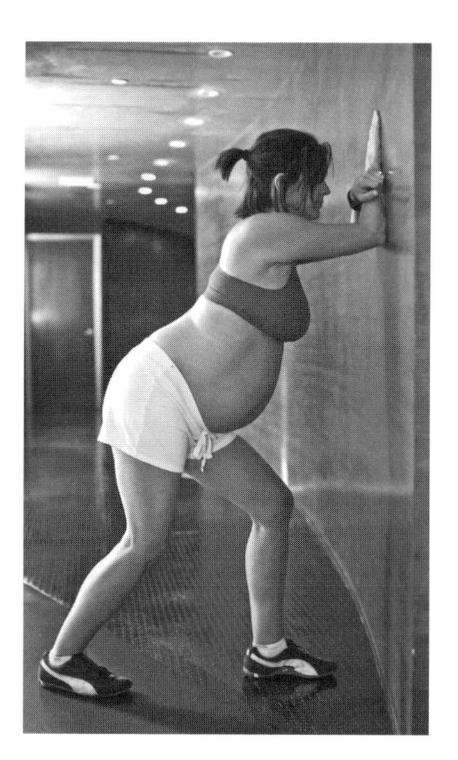

Calf stretches

You can also face a staircase and place the ball of your feet and toes on the bottom step. Drop one heel and feel the stretch in your calf. Hold for 30 seconds.

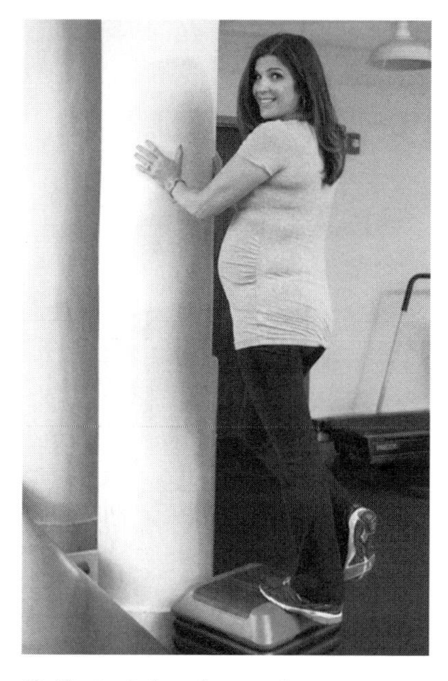

Calf stretch using a step

Magnesium and Leg Cramps

The use of magnesium supplements can help your night cramps. Eighty-six pregnant women participated in a 2012 study regarding the benefits of magnesium for leg cramps. Half the women took magnesium and the other half took a placebo. The results of this study show that an oral magnesium supplement can decrease the frequency and intensity of pregnancy-induced leg cramps. This was seen in half the women that took the supplement. Another study showed leg cramps are a common symptom in pregnancy and in patients with low serum levels of magnesium. A supplement could be helpful for these women.

And yet another study looked at magnesium levels in blood and urine in women who were taking oral magnesium supplements. It was concluded that magnesium levels don't elevate in the blood, as any extraneous amounts are eliminated in urine. So are they safe for everyone? As with any change in your diet or use of supplements, you should discuss it with your doctor or midwife.

Options that have not been proven to decrease calf cramps include compressive hosiery, calcium salts, analgesics, antiepileptic drugs, multivitamin and mineral supplements, quinine alone or with theophylline, sodium chloride, and stretching exercises. In fact, pregnant women are advised not to take quinine. Even though the research hasn't supported calf stretching as a definite cure for leg cramps, our patients have reported that it definitely helps.

We gave Jessica a ProStretch and advised her to stretch her calves at least twice a day, with one time being before she went to bed. This helped her for a week and she told us she did the happy pregnant dance. But unfortunately they came back. She started walking home from work, but that didn't help. She began drinking diluted Gatorade throughout the day. The extra electrolytes decreased the frequency of her cramps down to once each night. She elevated the end of her bed but was too uncomfortable sleeping like this so she lowered it. In the end, she ditched her heels and wore sneakers every day. She loved fashion and hated this last resort. The comfortable footwear decreased her leg cramps to every other night, so she felt better.

Pelvic Pain

Kelsey was your typical butt clencher. Always on the go, always had meetings and appointments, always looking at her watch. Not that all Type A personalities automatically qualify as butt clenchers, but they generally are the ones who have trouble relaxing. She came to see us for pelvic floor pain. She wanted her pregnancy to be perfect and she was already in pain, just a few weeks along.

What does it mean to be a butt clencher? It means that you constantly tighten (or "guard") your pelvic floor muscles, even when you don't need to. You need to tighten your pelvic floor muscles when you are trying to hold in your urine or gas. However, butt clenchers are either used to tensing all their muscles in the pelvis all the time *or* they are tensing all the time because they are in pain. People tend to guard or tighten their muscles when they are experiencing some pain in their pelvis, but some then don't remember how to let go and relax. And we say "butt clencher" because generally people just clench all the muscles in their pelvis, not just the pelvic floor muscles.

When most butt clenchers are told to relax, they generally respond with, "I am relaxed." They think that they are resting and have turned their muscles "off," but their muscles are still very much turned "on." When people have tightened muscles for a long time, they can develop pain in the muscles because of spasms and trigger points.

And yes, it may seem as if your entire pelvis can be hurting you all at once. Among all the relevant studies, pelvic pain can occur in up to 76 percent of all pregnancies. And this is because pelvic pain can occur in the front of the pelvis, in the back of the pelvis, on one side, or on both sides. It can be due to hormonal, traumatic, or mechanical factors. But if you use our tips for treatment, you'll be able to manage these symptoms and be able to get that nursery ready in no time.

What you can do

For Kelsey the first step was making her realize that she was clenching her muscles. We took away her appointment book, smartphone, watch, smartphone ear piece, mp3 player, and iPad, so she could focus on her body with minimal external stimulation. Kelsey had to first understand where exactly she was holding tension in her body and why. We used different techniques to improve her awareness. She closed her eyes and focused on each body part to see if it was relaxed. This helped her see that she was holding excess tension throughout her body, especially in her pelvis. We used biofeedback to help Kelsey actually see her muscle activity. This involved putting (pain-free) electrode stickers on her pelvic floor muscles, near her rectum. The electrodes were connected to our computer and she could see when her muscles were relaxed or contracted. She wasn't able to relax these muscles initially, but by the end of the first session we came up with a treatment plan involving several exercises to relax her pelvic floor muscles.

Apps to Relax

Yes, we talked about letting go of your electronic devices in order to focus on relaxing your tight muscles. However, your smartphone may actually come in handy for this purpose. There are many relaxation, visualization, and meditation apps that you can download. Many of these programs have reminder alerts and timers, so all of you busy bees need only to set aside a few minutes a day to relax. The best part about these apps is that they are free!

There are different techniques for relaxing the pelvic floor muscles. Besides learning how to relax and breathe properly, learning how to stretch these tight muscles is really important. The purpose of this next stretch is to lengthen the pelvic floor muscles. These muscles generally take on the brunt of pelvic tightness.

- Lie on your back and bring your knees up to your chest.
- Grab onto the inside of your ankles to increase the stretch. Make sure your knees are pointing outward and that your thighs are in a "V" position.
- Pull up on your ankles and feel the stretch in your perineal area (basically, your "crotch"). Hold this stretch for 30 seconds at least.
- Do two to three repetitions of this stretch.

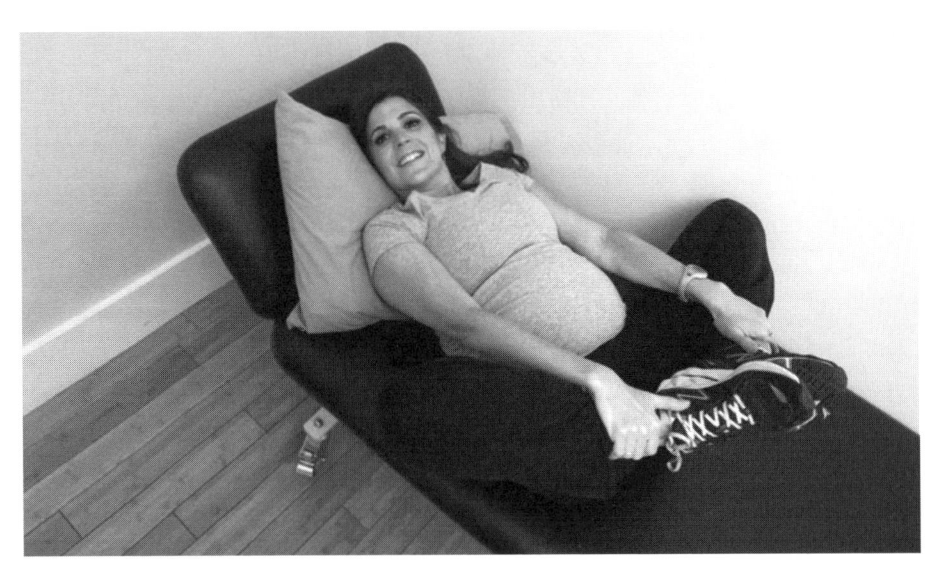

Pelvic floor stretch

You can also be super fancy and stretch two muscles at once! You have to have good balance to perform this next stretch, or you may end up on the floor, so please be careful. This next stretch is to lengthen both the hip flexors (the muscles in the front of your hip) as well as your hip extensors (the muscles in the back of your hip) at the same time.

- Lie on the edge of your bed hugging one knee to your chest and letting one leg hang off the bed.
- Grab onto the lower leg ankle and bring it toward your buttocks. Hold this stretch for 30 seconds.
- Do two to three repetitions.

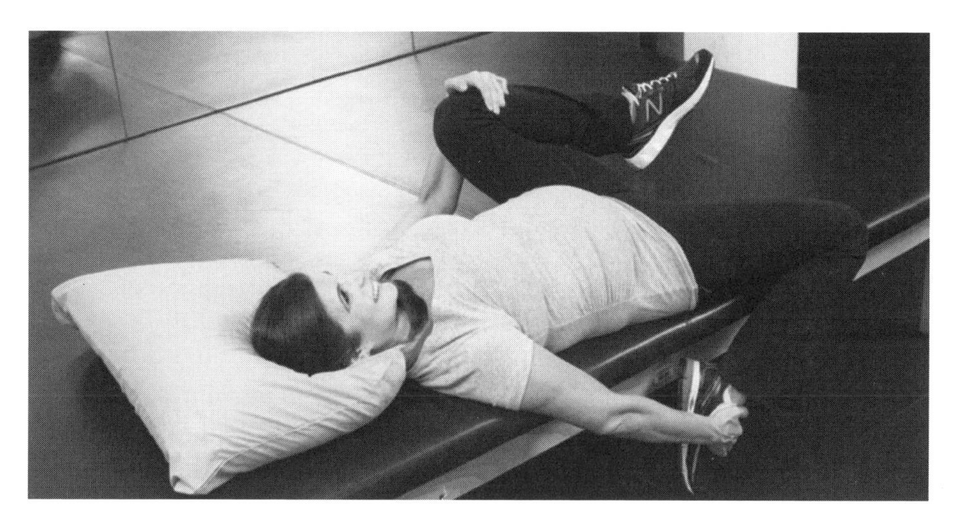

Hip flexor and hip extensor stretch

You can try stretching one muscle at a time (this is the stretch for just the hip extensors):

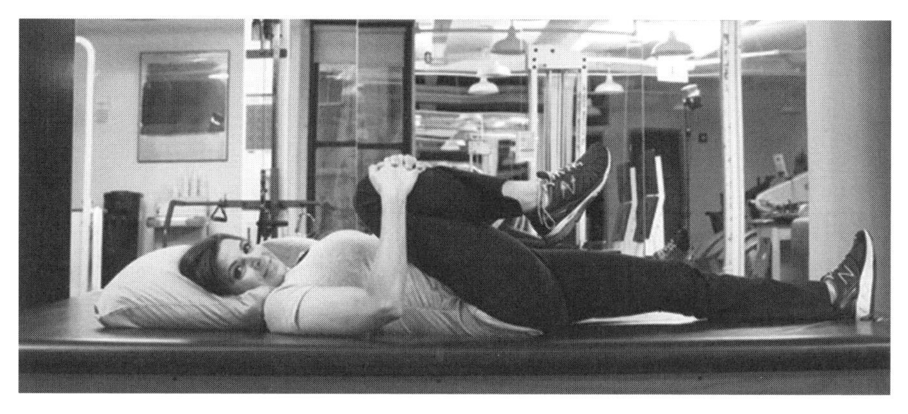

Gluteus maximus stretch

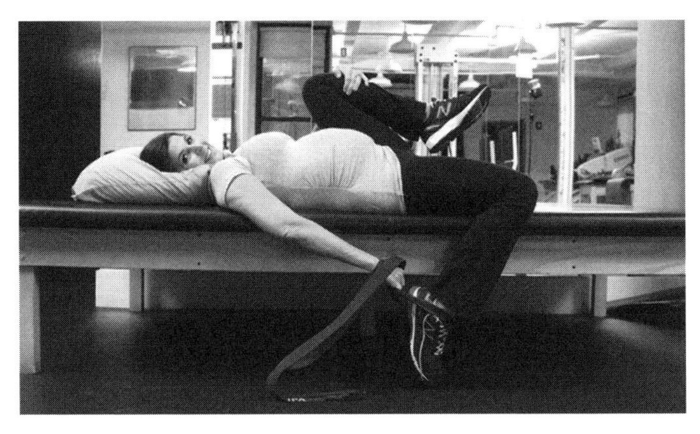

Combination hip flexor/hip extensor stretch using a strap

You can use a stretching strap to help you further stretch the hip flexors of your bottom leg.

When it's more than a tight pelvic floor

There are other problems that can occur when the bones in your pelvis separate, including upslips, outflares, subluxations, and muscle strains. Corrections will not be explained for these or other pathologies, as they need to be supervised by a physical therapist or other qualified health care provider. As with all exercises and treatments, please consult with your doctor or midwife before practicing them.

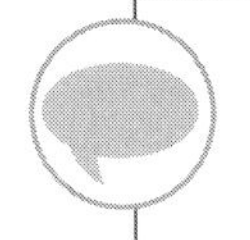

From Denise: I have suffered from pelvic pain throughout most of my life. I have suffered from pain due to endometriosis since I was a little girl. Once I understood my pain and that I was guarding and tightening my muscles due to this pain, I knew I needed to address this. I performed the stretches described above on a regular basis. I learned to relax my muscles and breathe more deeply and efficiently. These techniques have helped me tremendously. I continue to do them daily to avoid flare-ups. Remember: stretches, breathing, relaxation.

Pubic Symphysis Pain/Symphysis Pubis Dysfunction

Lilly came into the office during her eighth month of pregnancy. She was clutching the front of her pelvis and was walking very slowly. What was her problem? Besides knowing that she was going to push a watermelon out of her body? She had pubic symphysis pain (also called symphysis pubis dysfunction (SPD)). This pain began two months ago. Her partner helped her get in and out of bed. She was unable to sit in small chairs with the kindergartners she taught. Her school didn't have elevators and she needed help from a colleague to get up and down the stairs to reach her classroom. She asked her doctor to perform an early C-section, as she couldn't make it another month with so much pain. She felt and heard a lot of clicking and popping and thought her pelvis was falling apart when she walked/waddled.

The pubic symphysis is that spot in the front of your pelvis that lies right under your zipper of your pre-maternity pants. The two halves of your pelvis are held together by cartilage in the front; this "joint" is called the pubic symphysis.

As your pregnancy progresses, the cartilage separates slightly to allow the baby to grow, drop, and be delivered. This is a response to your increasing pregnancy. The problem here is that because the front of the pelvis is not fastened together with more bone, the cartilage can react to the hormone a little too much. This can cause the bones to separate more than they need to. The separation is only supposed to be as much as four to five millimeters (which is about 0.2 inches). With pregnancy, it will increase by two to three millimeters. However, if the separation is between 10 and 13 millimeters, you have a pubic symphysis separation or "pubic symphysis diastasis." Your separation is about half an inch. So what does this mean? PAIN! Pain from the misaligned pelvis can remain local or spread to the low back, groin, abdomen, inner thighs, and hips.

When the pubic symphysis softens to prepare for expansion, one side may shift. There are numerous culprits for this. Your baby may be spending more time on one side of the uterus. If you're carrying multiples, one baby may be larger and stressing one side more than the other. Or, your activities may favor one side, such as only holding a child or heavy bag on your left, to free up your dominant right arm. Even more simply, you might be stronger or tighter on one side, which will pull your pelvic bones into an unfavorable position.

Whatever the cause is, when your pelvis shifts, it can be very painful. We see this often in our physical therapy practices, but pregnant women are more susceptible when their pregnancy hormones are at their highest levels. To alleviate the pain we need to stabilize the pelvis so it does not move too much as you walk.

What you shouldn't do

- Walking lunges
- Walking up big hills
- Using gym equipment that forces your legs to move far apart in opposite directions (elliptical, steep incline on a treadmill, abductor machine)

Here are some labor positions to avoid if you have PSD:

- Giving birth on your back with legs in stirrups or on attendant's hips or shoulders
- Semi-sitting; this tends to force the baby's head against the pubic symphysis
- Second stage positions where the knees are pulled back toward the chest

What you can do

There are exercises you can do to stabilize your pelvis using your muscles. The muscles on the inside of your thigh are called the *adductors*. Your adductors connect also to the sides of your pubic symphysis. Strengthening your adductors will help keep your pubic symphysis stable.

This is one of the easiest exercises you can do to achieve this.

- Lie on your back with your knees bent and squeeze a pillow between your knees. Double up the pillow if it isn't plush enough to squeeze.
- Squeeze for five seconds (keep breathing!) and relax.
- Do two sets of 10.

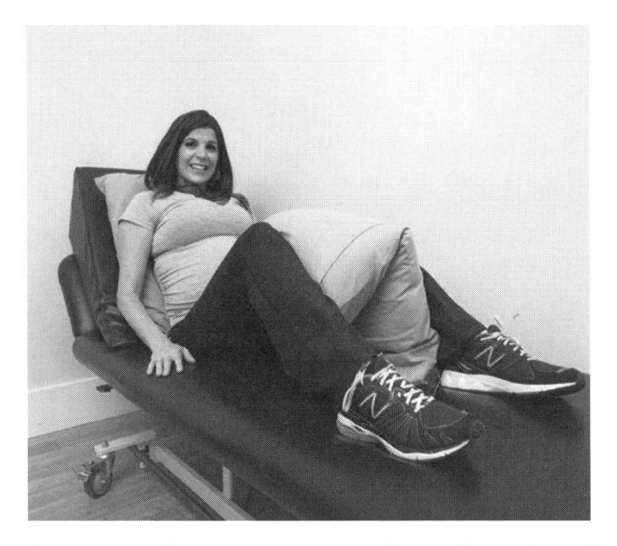

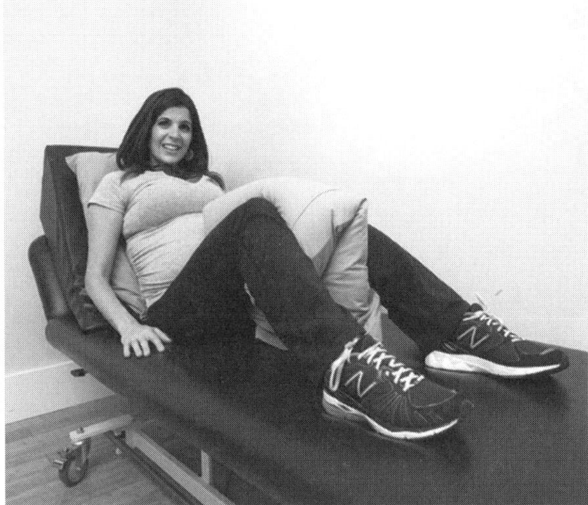

Pelvic stabilization exercises with a pillow: hip adduction

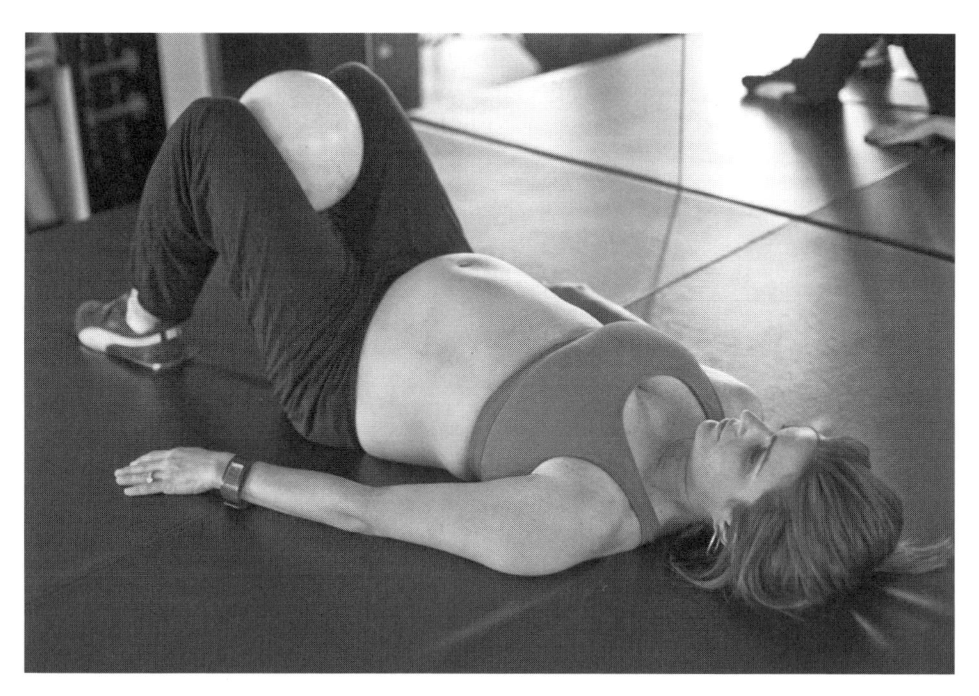

Pelvic stabilization exercises with a ball: hip adduction

You can also squeeze a small ball.

Or use a partner to help you with this exercise. Tell your partner to place his or her hands on the inside of your knees and resist you bringing your knees together. Your partner doesn't have to use Herculean force, just enough to equal your resistance.

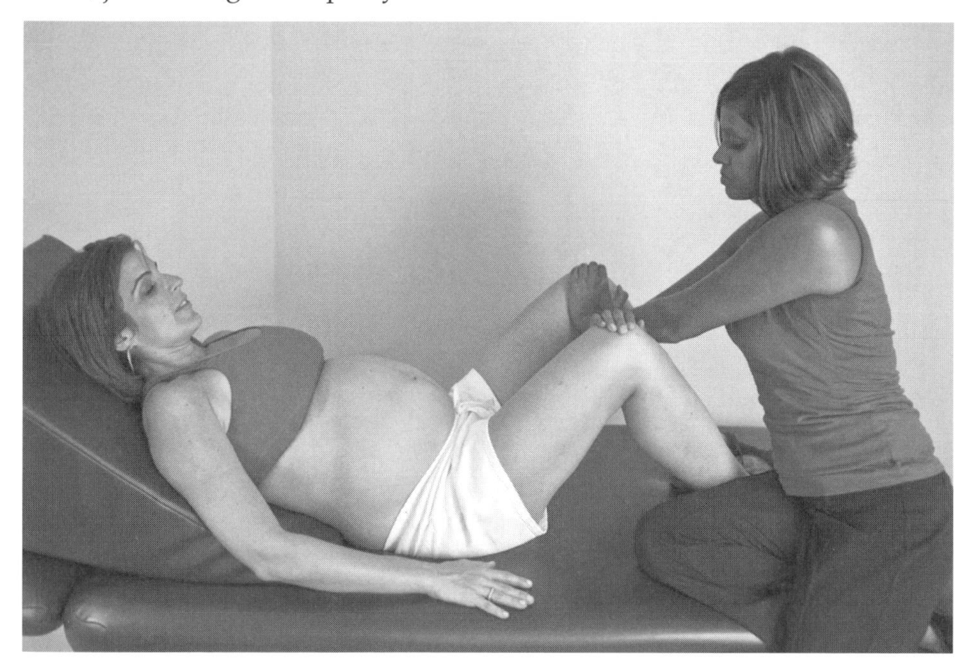

Partner-assisted pelvic stabilization exercises

You may sometimes feel discomfort in your pubic symphysis while getting up from your seat. One inconspicuous thing you can do is squeeze your purse in between your knees as you stand up. We're women so we're assuming you all have some kind of purse or backpack accessory with you. Squeezing your purse (or fist if you're traveling light) between your knees while you are getting up from a chair helps to stabilize your pubic symphysis because you are contracting those adductors again. It's a secret. No one knows you are doing it!

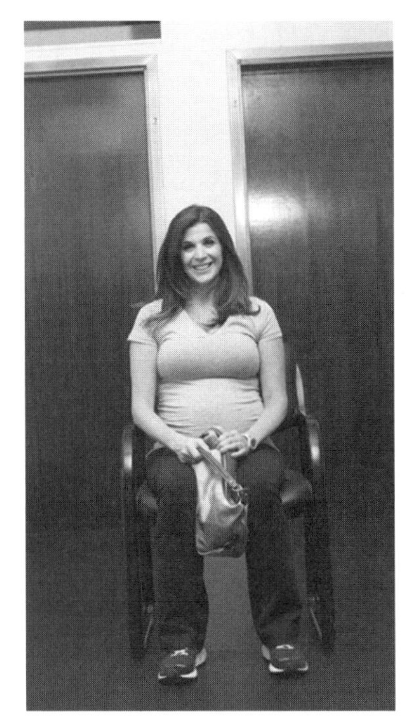
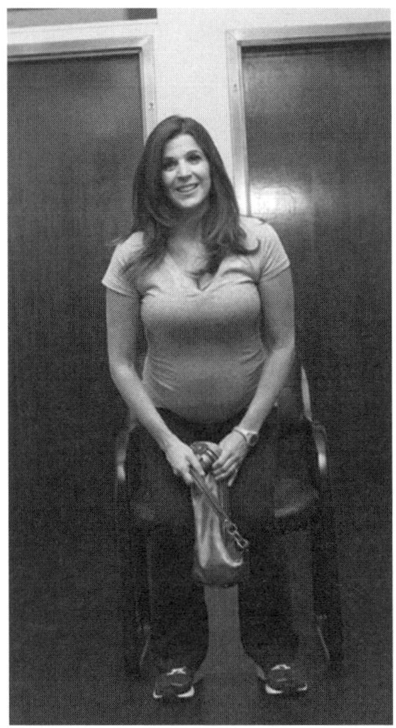
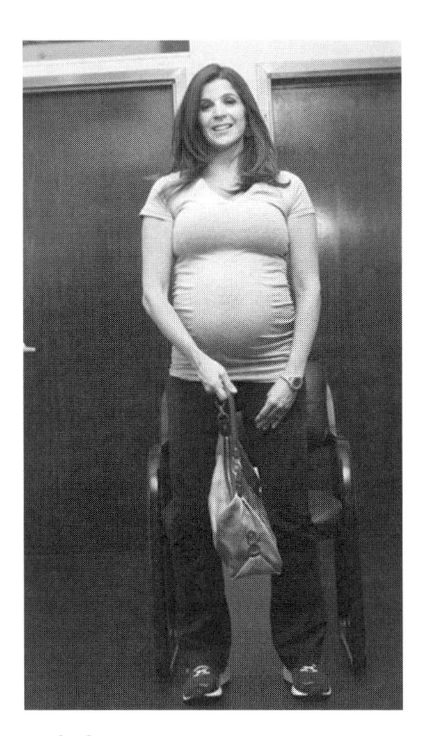

Using your purse to ease pubic symphysis pain while getting up from a chair

Similarly, this trick can be used to get in and out of a car. Instead of stepping into the front seat as you normally do, practice the following technique:

- Open the car door.
- Turn your body so you can sit on the seat with both feet on the ground.
- Contract your abdominals while supporting your body with both hands on your seat.
- Keep your knees together and swing both legs into the car. Your body moves with your legs so you are facing forward.

Reverse this to get out of your car.

- Open the car door.
- Contract your abdominals and support your body with your hands on the seat.
- Bring your legs onto the ground while keeping your knees together. Turn your body at the same time so you can step out of the car without straining your pelvis.
- Keep your knees together and stand up to exit the car.

Try to avoid driving large SUVs if possible. Unless you play for the WNBA (Women's National Basketball Association), it is often difficult to reach the driver's seat. Taking a wide step up into the driver's seat can further strain this painful area.

Getting into bed is a similar process.

- Sit down on your bed with both feet on the floor and your knees together.
- Engage your abdominal muscles.
- Use your hands to help you lower your head to your pillow as you bring your feet up to the bed. You should be lying on your *side* at this point with your bent knees together.
- Maintain your engaged abdominal muscles and roll to your back.

To get out of bed, reverse the steps.

- Engage your abdominal muscles.
- Roll to your side with your knees together.
- Use your hands to push your upper body up to a sitting position as you lower your feet to the ground. Keep your knees together as you stand up.

(Refer to the section on diastasis recti for additional pictures on how to get out of bed safely while easing the discomfort of your pubic symphysis. Just make sure you are squeezing something in between your knees as you are getting up. You can use a pillow.)

Another option for relieving pain in the pubic symphysis is to use a belt. These belts are normally used for sacroiliac pain (pain in the back of the pelvis), but they can also be used for pubic symphysis pain (pain in the front of the pelvis). If you are experiencing pubic symphysis pain, the belt just needs to be flipped around so that the compression is

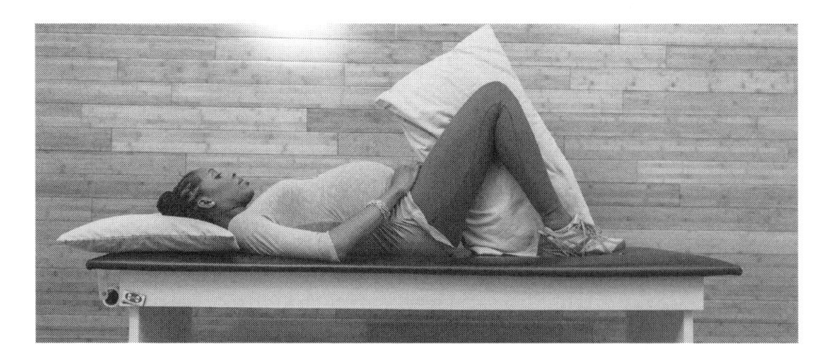

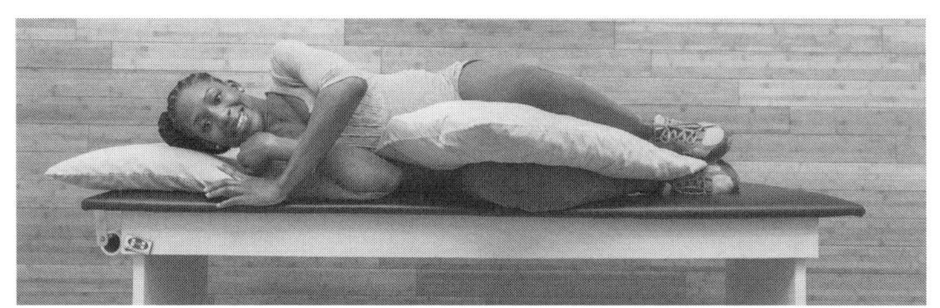

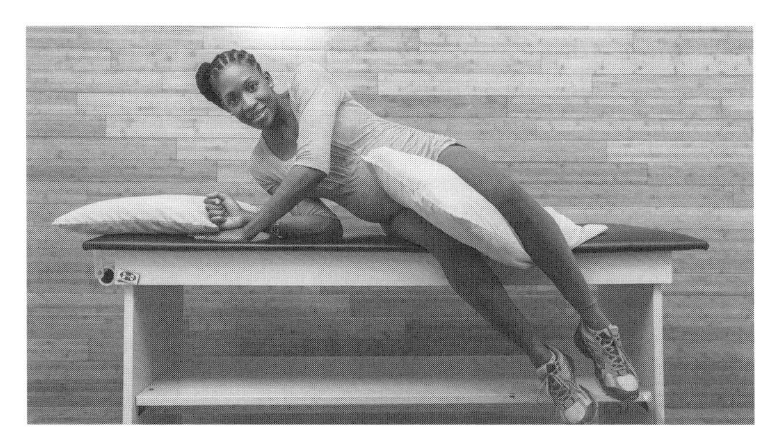

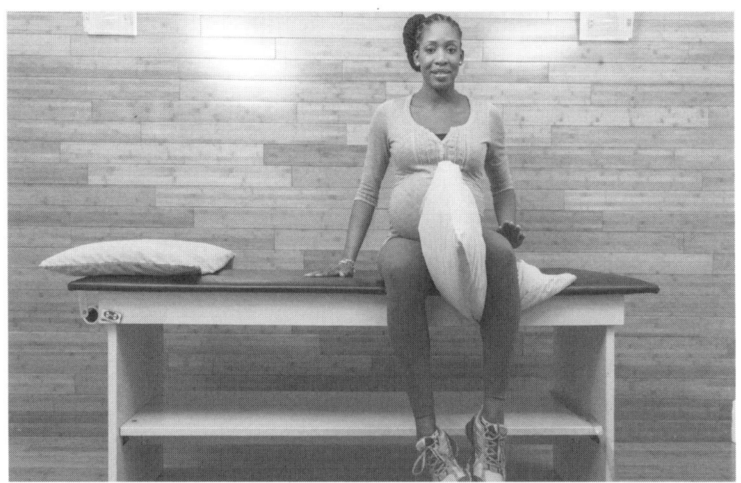

Getting out of bed safely with pubic symphysis pain using a pillow

applied forward to the front of your pelvis. These belts apply an external compressive force to help stabilize the pelvis and help you feel less "loose." It's important to apply these belts properly and in the correct spot. The belts should feel snug when they are applied correctly. Always consult with a physical therapist to make sure the belt is in the correct position, because they can cause great discomfort if they are positioned incorrectly.

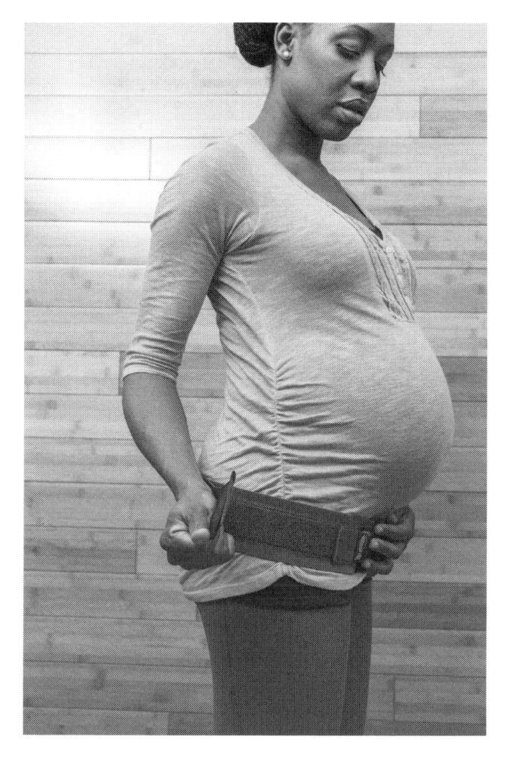

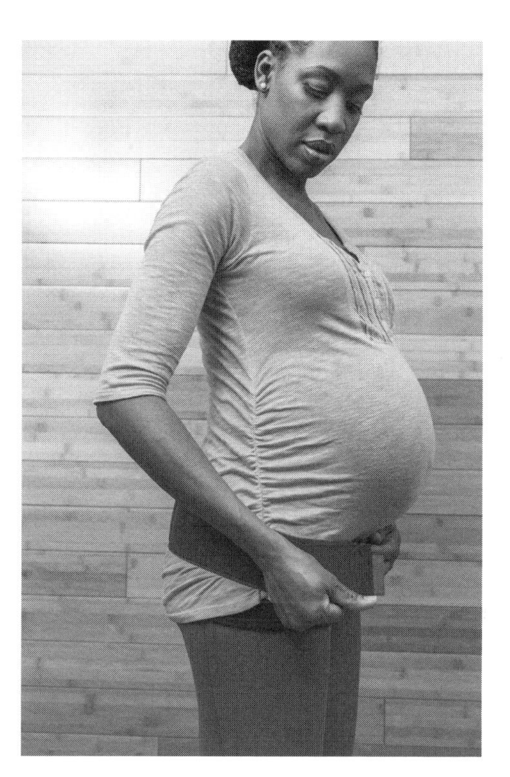

Pelvic belt for pubic symphysis pain

More Pubic Symphysis Relief

- Use a pillow or cushion between your knees when sleeping.
- Use a pillow under your tummy (in pregnancy) when sleeping (see section on sleeping pains).
- Keep your legs close together and parallel when moving, turning over in bed, getting in and out of cars, and so on (see previous section on how to get out of a car).
- Satin sheets or nightwear may make it easier to turn over in bed.
- When standing, stand with weight evenly distributed through both legs.

- Move slowly and without sudden movements—taking extra care not to slip or trip up.
- Sit down to put on underwear, socks, and pants.
- Avoid "straddle" movements.
- Avoid heavy lifting, twisting movements, and any other movements you know will hurt you—for example, vacuuming can often be a problem.
- Icepacks over the painful joint may reduce inflammation.
- Stretching the hamstrings can be helpful for sciatica. (See pages 60 to 61 for hamstring stretches.)
- Use some kind of pelvic support.
- If sex is uncomfortable for you, try different positions—for example, lying on your side with your back to your partner and a cushion between your knees.
- Swimming (not breaststroke) or walking in water can be helpful for some women. Others may find that the water's resistance puts too much stress on their joints. Do what works for you.
- In severe cases, use a walker, crutches, or a wheelchair. Your doctor can provide you with an application for a disabled parking card if necessary.
- Rest can be extremely helpful. However, it is best to keep as active as possible within the limits of your pain. Sometimes, gentle walking can reduce pain, but always take care not to overdo it. Listen to your body and your doctor or midwife.
- Ask for help. Friends and family are often your best resources. Talk to your doctor or medical professional about the possibility of organizing home help.

We advised Lilly to go up and down the stairs sideways, while holding on to the railing. This minimized her pain and allowed her to get to her classroom independently. She felt a significant improvement with the belt we gave her. It held her pelvic bones together so she no longer felt sharp pains if she moved too quickly. She did continue to take small steps, but with the brace she didn't hear the popping or feel as unstable. She did adductor strengthening exercises daily and used a thick pillow between her knees when getting out of bed. Her midwife was very careful during her delivery and she had her baby in a side-lying position to avoid excessive strain on her pelvis. She continued to wear the belt for two weeks postpartum and her symptoms resolved.

Sacroiliac Pain

Jane didn't know how or what she did wrong. She was just crossing the street during her lunch break when she experienced excruciating left low back pain. She could barely walk and getting into a cab would have been impossible had her colleague not been with her to help. She returned to work doubled over in pain. She was afraid to take any anti-inflammatories because she was 25 weeks pregnant. She made an appointment to see us that afternoon. She has a history of low back pain, but had been pain-free for over a year.

This is a common area in which to have pain during pregnancy. The sacrum is a large vertebra at the base of your spine, just above your tail bone. The ilia are the large bones in your pelvic girdle. If you put your hands on your waist (or what used to be your waist) and slide them down, you'll find these bones. The sacrum and the ilia form joints on both sides of your low back, connected by strong ligaments. These joints are usually sturdy, but nothing is immune to the overpowering pregnancy hormones. The hormones relax your pelvic joints so the bones can expand and your baby can descend. This system usually works, but it isn't perfect.

How Do You Know If You Have a Problem at Your Sacroiliac Joint?

You may experience the following:

- Pain in your low back, just above your butt, and off to either side.
- Swelling and discomfort when you touch this area.
- A sense of being out of alignment in your pelvis and low back.
- Pain can radiate into your butt, groin, legs, or low back.
- Limited motion in flexing, turning, or extending your trunk.
- Clicking or catching sensation in your low back when you try to get out of a chair or in/out of a car.
- Pain and difficulty putting on socks or pants on one side.

What you can do

Please contact your doctor or midwife if you are having these symptoms and ask for a physical therapy referral. Also, ask for permission to wear a sacroiliac belt. As painful as sacroiliac dysfunction is, this is one condition we don't recommend you try to treat yourself. Because your pelvis is made up of many parts, it can shift in many ways. One side can shift or rotate forward or backward. Or it can shift upwards or downwards. You may start to feel crooked and unbalanced. A physical therapist can evaluate you and treat you safely while you're pregnant. Until you can see someone, we have some suggestions to help manage your pain.

Wear a sacroiliac belt

This belt improves your pelvic stability, which can decrease your pain until you are further evaluated. We like the Serola Sacroiliac Belt.

To determine which size to get, refer to the sizing chart on the www.serola.net website. You can also check out the website to see a video on how to apply the belt.

Refer to the section on pubic symphysis pain (page 46) for more information on pelvic belts.

Bridging exercise

Refer to page 3 in the section on low back pain for instructions and pictures of bridging.

Hip rotator strengthening exercises

There are other muscles you should strengthen to stabilize your pelvis. These muscles, your hip rotators, go from your butt to your outer thigh. You can strengthen them using a resistance band or your partner.

- Tie the band around your knees while you are lying on your back with your knees bent. Make sure that your feet and knees are together and that the band is tied snug around your knees.
- Separate your knees against the resistance of the band and hold that position for three seconds (keep breathing!).
- Then relax and return to the starting position. You don't have to pull your knees apart too far because you don't want to stress the pubic symphysis.
- Do two sets of 10 and then relax.

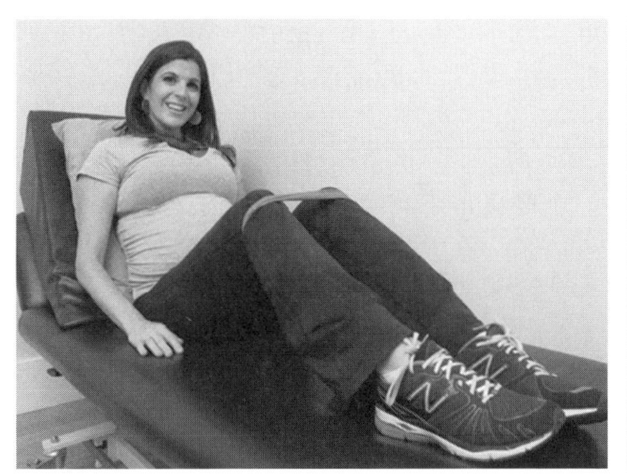
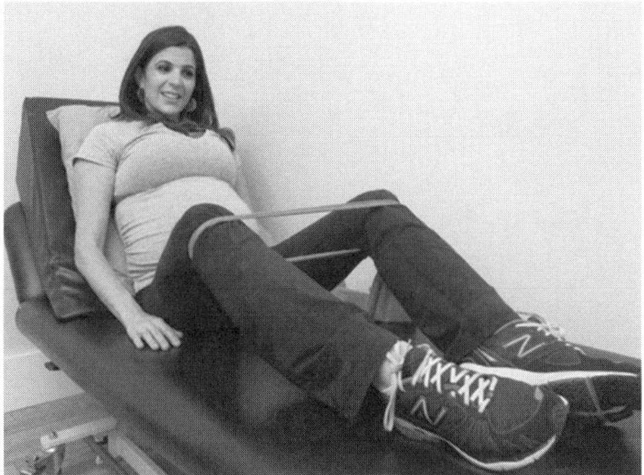

Pelvic stabilization exercises

Or you can use a partner for this exercise. Tell your partner to place his or her hands on the outside of your knees. You can push your knees outward against the resistance of your partner's hands and hold for two to three seconds. Push enough to meet your partner's resistance and don't separate your knees too far. Remember, you don't want to stress the pubic symphysis.

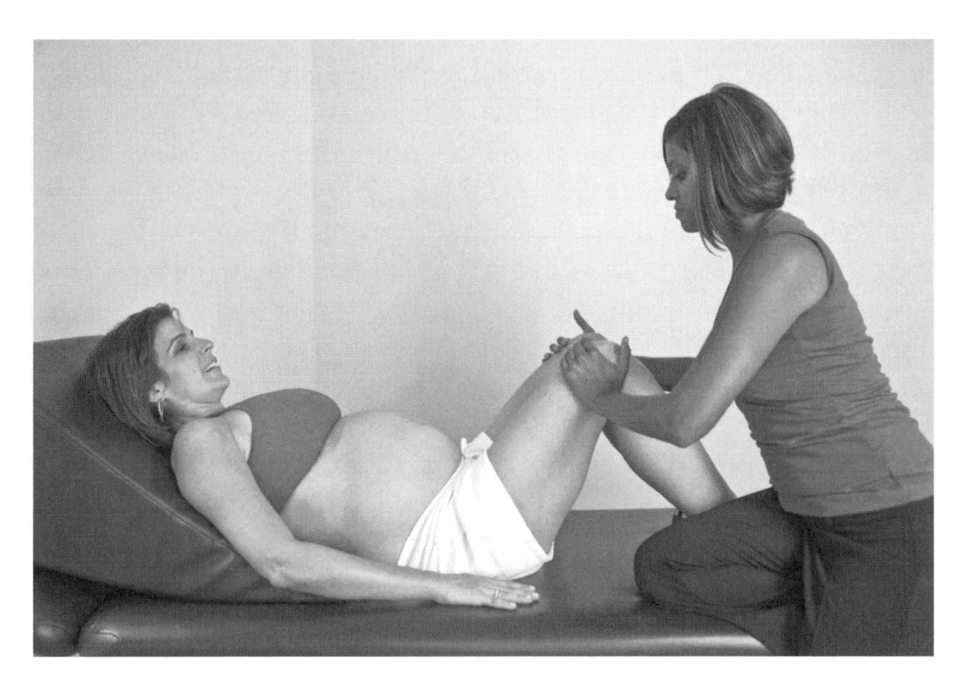

Pelvic stabilization exercises

Jane's acute pain resolved quickly. Her original pain at the back of her pelvis was corrected with some manual therapy and a stabilizing belt. This held her pelvic bones in the corrected position. She wore the belt every day, as she was afraid of another flare-up. She added some core strengthening exercises to her gym program and modified other components. She stopped doing lunges, single leg strengthening exercises, and high impact exercises for the remainder of her pregnancy. As she got stronger and less apprehensive, she weaned herself off the belt.

Sciatica

Sarah didn't know who to turn to. She was told this was a "pregnancy condition" and her pain would subside after she delivered. She was only six months pregnant and couldn't sit at her desk without pain radiating into her butt and down the outside of her right leg. She couldn't sleep without pain and the severity was worsening throughout her pregnancy. She was frustrated and tired of always being in pain.

Another pain in the ass! How many can we have? Too many, apparently. What is sciatica? It sounds like something emerging from Frankenstein's lab. And it can certainly feel like a monster has taken over your leg. One patient described it as "electricity spreading down the back of my leg." Other days it feels like someone is poking your butt cheek.

Why does this happen? The sciatic nerve is a big nerve—really big. It is the longest and widest single nerve in the body. No wonder it gets into so much trouble. It comprises five nerves from your lower spine that come together and travel down the leg into the foot. It can easily get pinched in different areas on its way down the back of the leg. The nerve can get pinched by a disc in the spine or a muscle in the hips. This can cause pain starting from the low back or from the buttock. Damage to this nerve can cause muscle weakness in the leg or foot, pins and needles sensation, pain, and difficulty walking.

What you can do

The sciatic nerve can get pinched in your piriformis muscle, a muscle in each butt cheek. This can result in pain or tingling in your butt and down your leg. Your piriformis muscle is generally a tight muscle because it is in a shortened position whenever you are sitting. Stretching the piriformis muscle may seem a little complicated, but will feel great when you do. You'll have to turn yourself into a bit of a pretzel. Let's start with the right leg.

- Lie on your back and bend your left knee.
- Place the outside of your right ankle on top of the left knee.
- Now, reach behind your left thigh and bring your leg in close to your chest. If it is too hard, ask your partner for some assistance. He or she can help bring your left knee to your chest, which will stretch your right butt muscles. Hold this stretch for 30 seconds.
- Repeat the stretch two to three times on each side.

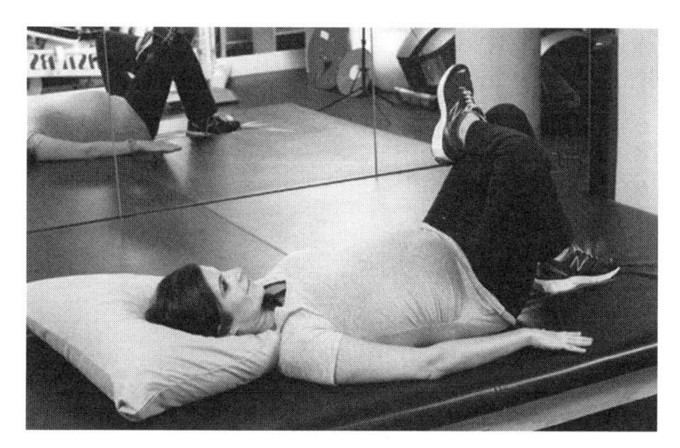

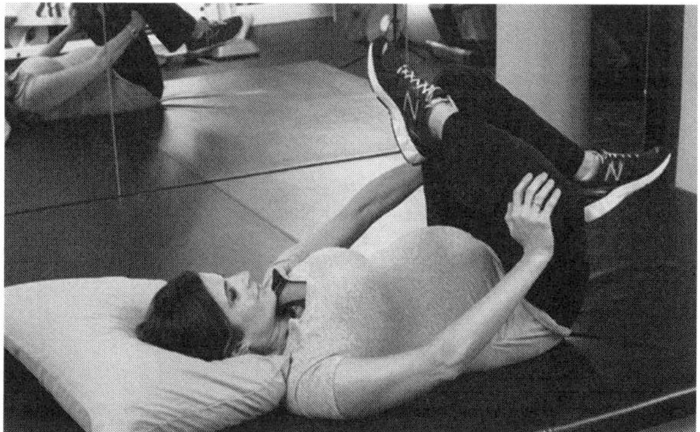

Stretching of the piriformis muscle

You can also have a partner help you stretch your piriformis muscle if your belly is getting in the way. Make sure your partner stretches you slowly and gently.

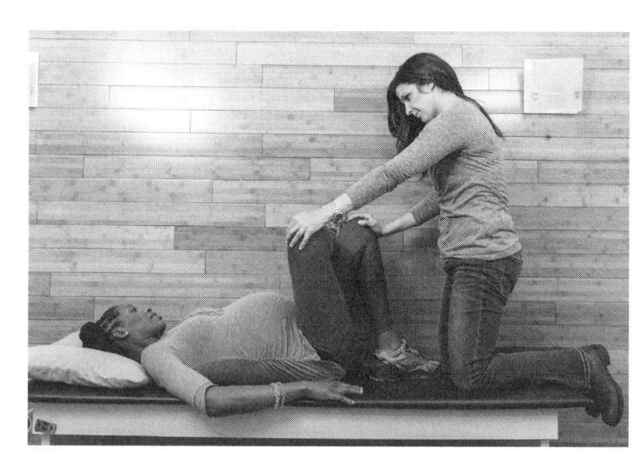

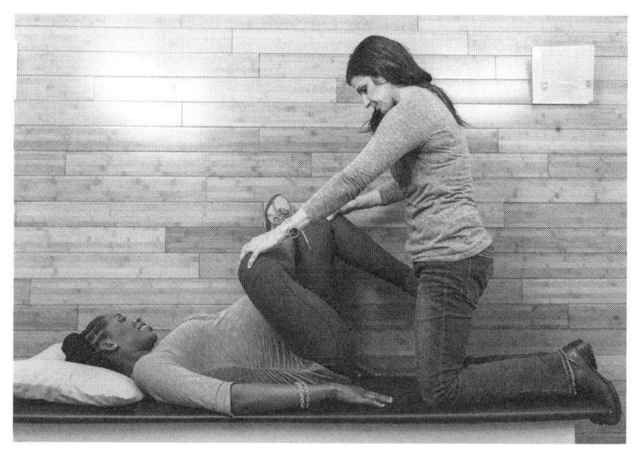

Partner stretch for piriformis muscle

If you have a foam roller, you can also try rolling out the tension in your piriformis.

- Position the foam roller perpendicular to your body on the floor.
- Sit on the foam roller and lean back with your hands on the floor behind you. Shift your weight onto one butt cheek.
- Take the leg of the side that you just shifted your weight onto and cross it over the opposite side.
- Now roll your butt cheek back and forth over the foam roller. In this position you should feel your hip rotator muscles more exposed. Roll back and forth until you feel a little easing of the tension in your bum. Repeat as often as you like.

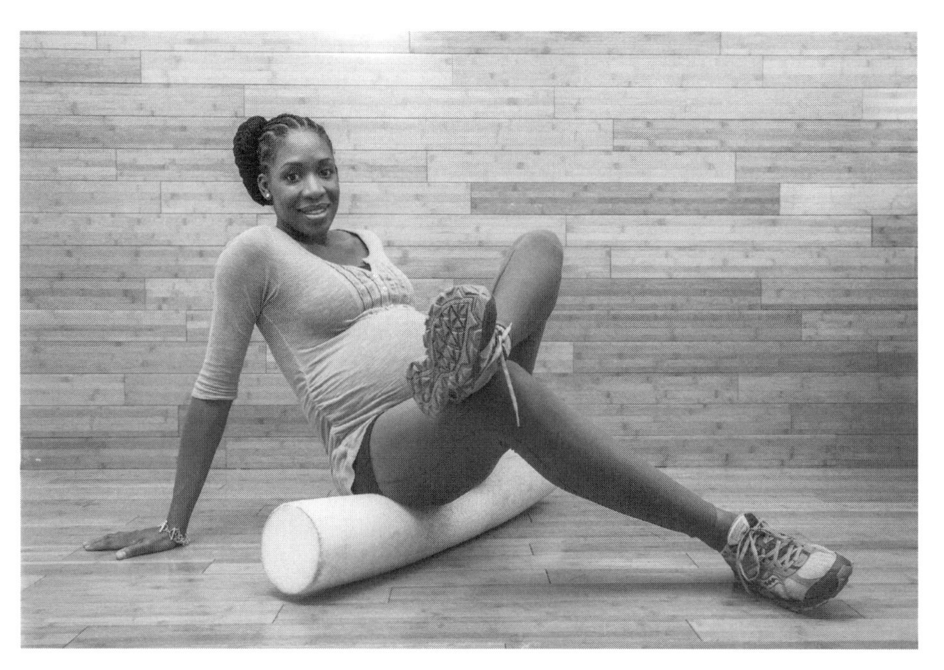

Foam rolling piriformis muscle

Another contributing factor to developing sciatica is having tight hamstrings. Your hamstrings start at the bottom of your butt and end behind your knee. When people have radiating pain down the back of the leg, they typically avoid taking big steps or moving the hamstring muscle through its full range of motion in order to avoid pain. This guarding can increase the tightness and the pain in the back of the leg. Also, the hamstrings are in a shortened position when you are sitting, so they have a tendency to become tight.

This stretch can also be done on your back. You may need a resistance band, belt, or stretching strap.

- Lift one leg straight up into the air and either grab onto the leg to increase the stretch or loop a band/belt/strap onto your foot to increase the stretch.
- Pull your leg toward your head and feel a lengthening of the muscle in the back of your leg. Hold this stretch for 30 seconds and repeat two to three times. Relax and then switch sides.
- If you are unable to do this yourself, ask your partner. Just make sure he or she stretches you slowly. Your tight muscles won't relax if the stretch is too aggressive.

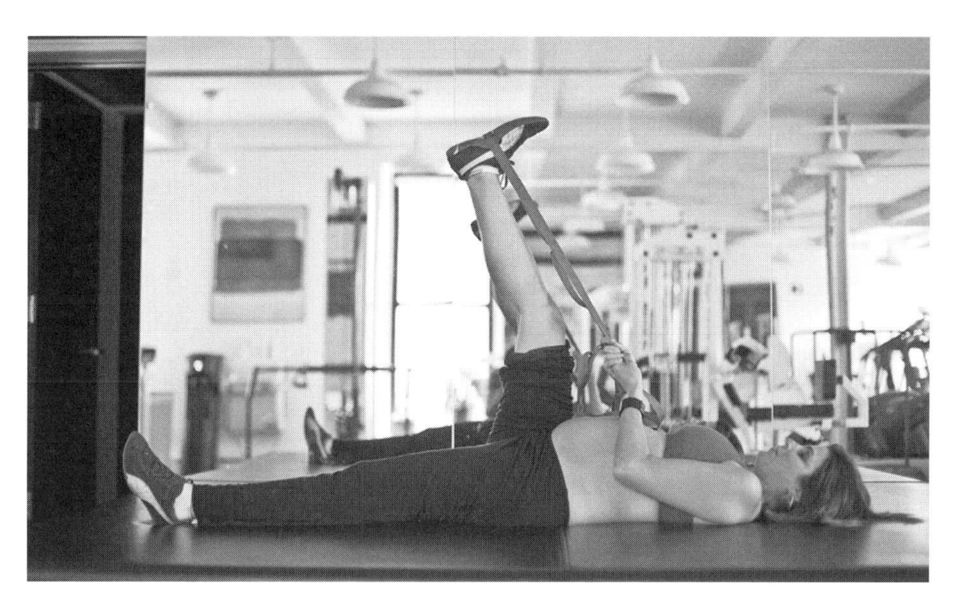

Hamstring stretch

Along with stretching the muscles, you may benefit from stretching the nerves. This is called nerve gliding or nerve flossing. The sciatic nerve travels along a path that takes it through muscles, between bones, and through some tight areas, as it travels down your legs from your spine. If it gets entrapped, there will be inflammation, pain, decreased blood flow, and difficulty moving. The pain is coming from pressure on the nerve, so additional massage or foam rolling won't help it. In fact, it will make it worse.

There are several areas where it can get entrapped, such as your butt muscles, deep thigh muscles, inner thigh muscles, or lower in your leg.

The sciatic nerve has the ability to stretch five inches, which is necessary for your legs to move freely. Think about bending forward toward the floor. If your sciatic nerve is restricted and it can't stretch with the surrounding muscles, you will have pain in that spot and you won't be able to move very far.

How do you know if your sciatic nerve is impinged? There is an easy test.

- Lie on your back with your legs straight. You can do this on your bed or floor.
- Using your hands, slowly bring one knee to your chest and attempt to straighten your knee. Stop when you feel a strong stretch.
- Once you accomplish this, attempt to bring the top of your foot toward your shin and hold it for five seconds. If you don't have any sciatic nerve restriction, you will feel a muscular stretch in your calf, behind your knee, or behind your thigh.
- While holding this position, bring your chin to your chest for five seconds. Your symptoms shouldn't change.

If you do have sciatic nerve entrapment, you will feel pain at the area where it is entrapped. You may feel sharp shooting pain in your leg or back. Repeat on the other leg so you can see if there is a difference in symptoms.

What should you do if your test is positive? Time for nerve gliding. You want to "floss" the nerve.

- While lying on your back, use a strap to hold up your leg (or you can use your hands if that is comfortable for you).
- Raise your leg high enough to elicit a gentle stretch behind your leg, but no pain.
- Point and flex your foot 20 times at this height (as if you are pushing a pedal). You will feel your pain intensify and lessen as you do this, with it feeling worse as your foot is brought toward your shin and less as you point it away. Your symptoms will be strong initially, but should lessen as the sciatic nerve loosens. When this happens, you will slowly be able to raise your leg higher. This should be a slow process.

If it feels less painful, try stretching your leg an inch higher to increase the nerve stretch and then relax it for several hours. Practice this nerve gliding for two minutes, twice a day. This isn't a lot of time—probably not enough time to listen to your favorite song—but it works.

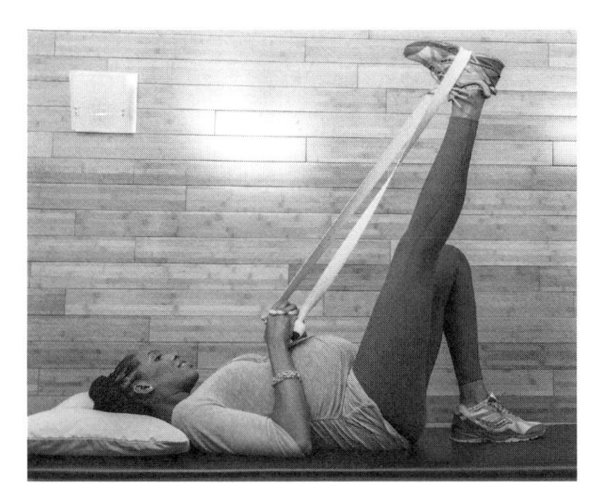

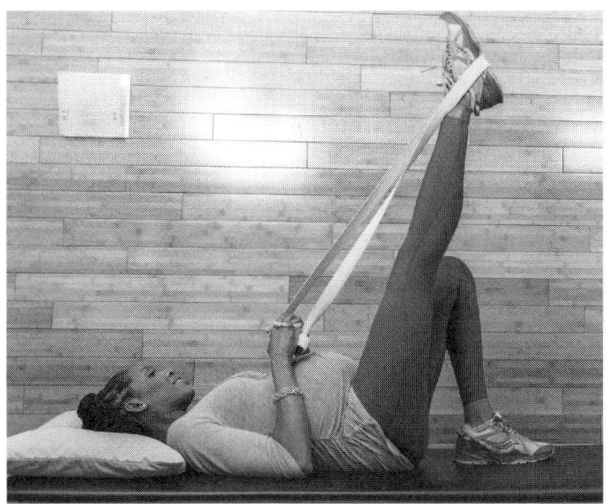

Nerve gliding

More Tips for Relieving Sciatica

- Wear flat shoes.
- Lie on pain-free side to release pressure in nerve.
- Work on posture.
- Wear maternity support to lift uterus.

Sarah survived her third trimester. She felt the most relief from wearing a maternity support. It lifted her uterus and relieved some pressure into her leg. Before going to sleep, she sat up in her bed with a heating pad on her low back/ butt (at the lowest setting) for 10 minutes. This soothed her pain and allowed her time to catch up on gossip magazines. Her partner helped her stretch her tight butt muscles. This was initially painful, but felt better each time.

Separated Abdominal Muscles (Diastasis Recti)

Giovanna said during her first pregnancy she didn't show until she was four months pregnant. By her fourth pregnancy, she was showing before she even peed on a stick. She said it looked like there was "a baguette" on her abdomen when she got out of bed in the morning. Her back pain was worsening as her pregnancy progressed. She was frequently asked if she was having twins. When she said she wasn't, the next question was, "Are you having triplets?" She was just too large for people to accept there was one baby in there.

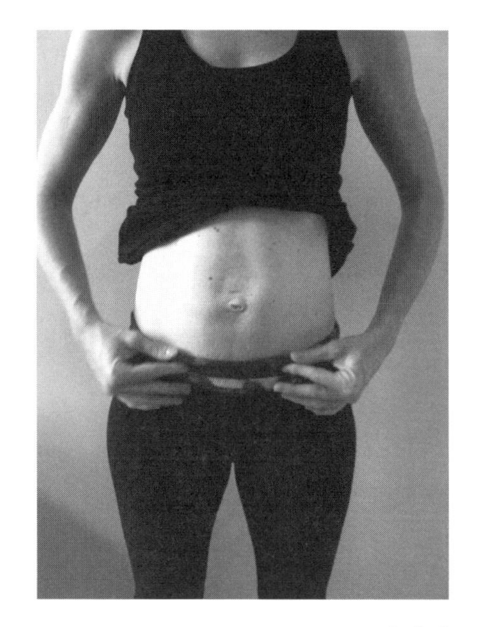

Has your belly button popped out? Is this supposed to happen? No, this shouldn't happen. You probably developed a diastasis recti of your abdominals. This is a common condition, and it can be prevented or corrected with the right program.

A diastasis occurs when your superficial abdominal muscles along your midline separate. Picture the ideal six-pack muscles separating into two three-packs. This can happen under many circumstances, including rapid weight gain, a growing uterus (especially when carrying multiples), excessive and incorrect abdominal work, and surgeries. It could also be a congenital condition that has been unknown until now.

The woman in this picture gained over half her body weight during her pregnancy. Because she is thin, her separated abdominal muscles are visible. She saw a doctor when she saw her organs "bulging" through her abdomen when she sat up.

Anatomy Lesson

There are four layers of abdominal muscles.

The deepest muscles are your transversus abdominis. They originate along the sides of your body and attach at the center of your abdomen, from your breastbone down to your pelvis. They are often called the "corset muscle" to describe the orientation of their muscle fibers wrapping around your core. Their main functions are to stabilize your trunk and pelvis and maintain internal abdominal pressure. When strong, these muscles make you look better in your swimsuit as they flatten your belly, if you need an aesthetic motivator.

The middle layers are your external and internal oblique muscles. These muscles cover a lot of abdominal territory, but to put it simply, they are located on the sides of your abdomen, from your low back and ribs, to the middle of your abdomen and pelvis. The internal obliques lie behind the external obliques. They work together to twist and sidebend your trunk. They also work in conjunction with your diaphragm to help you breathe.

The most superficial muscles are your rectus abdominis. Like your transverse abdominis, they cover the front of your core, from your breastbone down to your pelvis. When well-defined in non-pregnant individuals with low body fat, these two muscles make up your dreamy "six pack." The main functions of the rectus abdominis are to flex your trunk forward, stabilize your pelvis, and help you breathe.

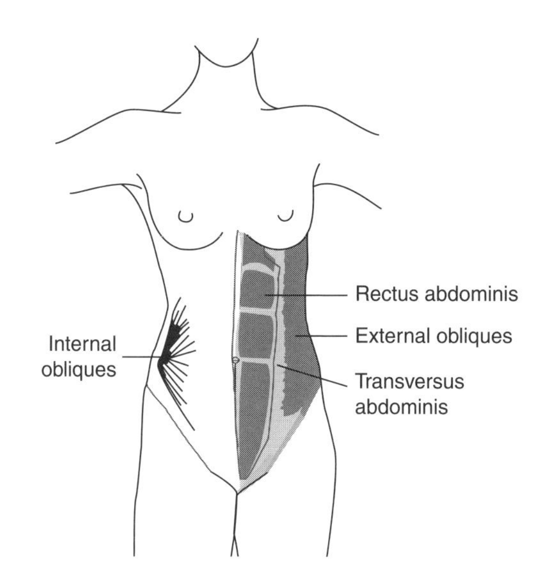

Of all your abdominal muscles, the transverse abdominis are usually the weakest, and most neglected. When they're strong, they hold your abdominal contents in place and support your spine. When they're too weak, your belly will protrude, because now connective tissue is supporting your organs instead of a strong muscular abdominal wall. Other muscles will have to compensate to give you the stability you need. This often results in low back pain, poor posture, impaired digestion, and abdominal discomfort.

Curious how these often ignored muscles work? Try contracting them. Pull your belly button back toward your spine as if you're trying to button your skinniest jeans. Feel them? Now it's time to get acquainted with them, as you should be exercising them throughout the day. Strong transverse abdominis muscles are the secret to preventing and closing a diastasis.

Who Are These Women With Diastases?

If women are pregnant, they might see a bulge along the midline of their bellies when they sit up from leaning back. Their belly button may also have popped out. They may be showing early in the pregnancy too. If they already gave birth, they may still look about five months pregnant while their baby is learning how to walk. They may have lost all their baby weight, but they still have a protruding abdomen, can't fit into their clothes, and are insulted every time someone offers them a seat on the subway. As physical therapists in New York City, we see these women daily, both on the streets and in our offices.

Diastasis Recti Risk Factors

- Older women (older than 33 years)
- Multiparity
- Multiple gestation
- Carrying a larger baby (>3,636 gram or 8 pounds)
- Greater weight gain (>35 lb)
- Birth by Cesarean section

We've had several patients tell us about their painful plastic surgeries to repair their abdominal muscles. These women were strong and fit with toned muscles everywhere. So why did they have such problems with their abdominals? Their stories were all very similar. They did lots of crunches while they were small enough during their first trimesters. Then they switched to planks and exercises on their hands and knees to accommodate their growing bellies. After delivery, they resumed sit-ups and aggressive abdominal work to flatten their stomachs. As they burned calories galore and shed pounds everywhere, their protruding bellies didn't improve. Countless hours and dollars were spent on personal trainers and boot camp classes. Their last resort was sadly met at the plastic surgeon's office. So, we often hear that they wish they had known the right exercises to do while they were pregnant.

What you shouldn't do

- Crunches, sit-ups, and exercises where both your shoulders and legs are off the ground (bicycle crunches) should be avoided, as you can't engage your transverse abdominis muscles with these exercises. You can create a diastasis or make an existing separation worse. If you do these exercises, you may see your abdominal muscles push out as you lift your shoulders off the floor. It will look like half a football bulging out of your abdomen near your belly button. Or, you may see a gap between the muscles, which didn't use to be there. *You don't want either of these scenarios.*

- Exercises in the plank position (push-up position) or on your hands and knees should also be avoided. If the connective tissue is too thin and your muscles are separated, you could cause a diastasis or make your diastasis worse by exercising on your hands and knees. Why? Because the weight of your baby and all your organs are now pressing on the weak connective tissue in this position. You may be engaging your core muscles, but if they're separated, they're not helping you where you need it. You want to *avoid* this position.

Now picture the fight between weak abdominal muscles and a growing uterus. Yes, your baby wins from the very start. You want your muscles to stretch to accommodate your growing uterus, not the connective tissue in between.

Healthy connective tissue between the two halves of your abdominal muscles should be two centimeters wide above your belly button and half the distance below. Two centimeters is about the diameter of a penny. Are you seeing a wider gap than that? Don't be surprised if you are. Much of the research on diastases is no longer current. However,

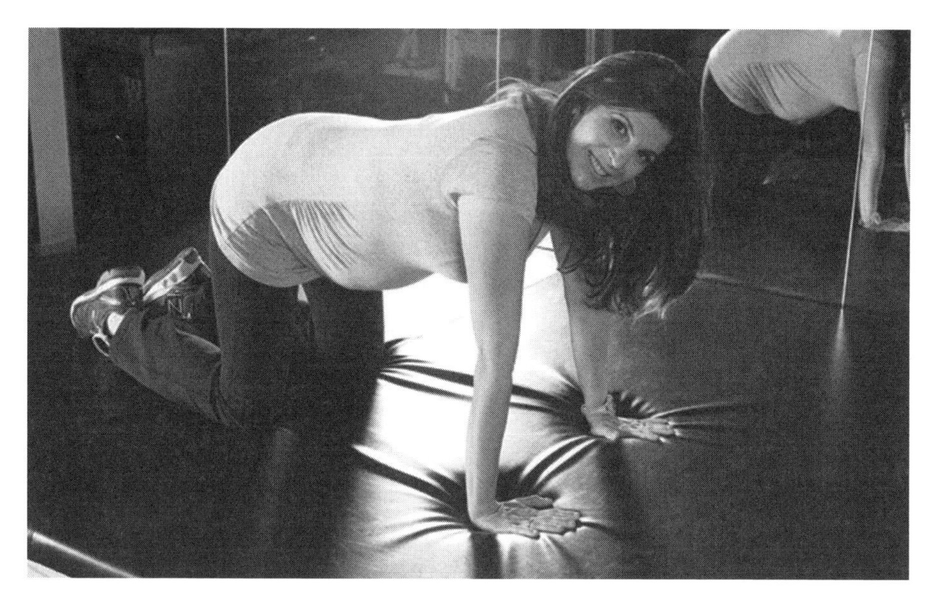

AVOID positions/exercises on your hands and knees.

when it was conducted in the 1980s, it showed that 66 percent of women had diastases in their third trimesters, 53 percent of these women continued to have a diastasis immediately postpartum, and 36 percent remained abnormally wide at five to seven weeks postpartum. We see much higher numbers than these in our practices. Many diastases aren't diagnosed. When women see physical therapists for their low back pain, pelvic pain, or pelvic dysfunction, they are often treated for a diastasis recti. Their weakened core can contribute to other painful and problematic diagnoses.

Could you be one of these women? Is the connective tissue near your belly button wider than a penny?

How to check for diastasis

A diastasis can be checked both during and after pregnancy. The object is to determine how many fingers will fit in the space between the two outermost abdominal muscles and how deep they penetrate.

Five easy steps

1. Lie on your back with your knees bent.
2. Place your middle three fingers in your belly button pointing in the direction of your toes.
3. Relax your abdominal muscles and lift your head. If you are holding your abdominal muscles in as you check it will give you a false reading as this will make the diastasis appear smaller.

4. Check yourself when you first start feeling the muscles come together. Raise and lower your head a few times so you can feel how the muscles work.

5. Use your fingers to feel both the depth and width of the separation. You may use as little as two to three fingers or need to use all 10 to feel the muscle borders. If it looks like half a football is trying to exit your core when you sit up, this means your diastasis is large and you will need two hands to measure it.

After testing yourself, if you think you may have a diastasis, you should contact a women's health physical therapist or a fitness professional who specializes in diastases. He or she will examine the integrity of your connective tissue between the separated muscles, measure the severity of the diastasis, and teach you the protocol to correct it. You will learn how to correctly strengthen your transverse abdominis. If you are unable to see a specialist, there are several videos you can watch to help you correct your diastasis on your own. One video we recommend is from Julie Tupler, RN. Her diastasis videos are available at www.diastasisrehab.com. Tupler Technique® Perfect Pushing® is designed for pregnant women to prevent and treat their diastases.

Please don't worry if you do develop a diastasis during your pregnancy. You're not sentenced to live through the rest of your pregnancy (or life for that matter) feeling like your muscles were put through a paper shredder. We've had many patients successfully prevent and treat their diastases. This abdominal tissue was strong at one point. You can get it strong again by working the right muscles and being careful with your movements. Treating and preventing a diastasis while pregnant may prevent you from having to deal with it later on. And remember, your belly button should not pop out! That's a sign of weak abdominal tissue.

How to Prevent a Diastasis

Transverse abdominal exercises

Here is an exercise you can do to help strengthen your transversus abdominis muscle.

- Sit in a chair with your feet touching the floor.
- Sit up straight and remember to keep breathing while you are performing these exercises. It's easy to want to hold your breath while you are contracting your abdominal muscles. Keep breathing!
- Practice pulling your belly button back toward your spine. Make sure that the only thing moving is your belly button. Don't rock your

pelvis back along with the movement. Don't arch or flatten your back. Don't raise or lower your shoulders. And don't bring your chest forward and back. These are all cheating techniques our patients try when their abdominals are too weak.

- If you feel like you can contract your abdominal muscle and still keep breathing, then try lifting one foot off the floor. Hold it off the floor while contracting your abdominal muscles for two to three seconds.
- Place that foot on the floor and lift the opposite leg. Repeat 10 times.
- You can also try lifting your opposite arm up at the same time.

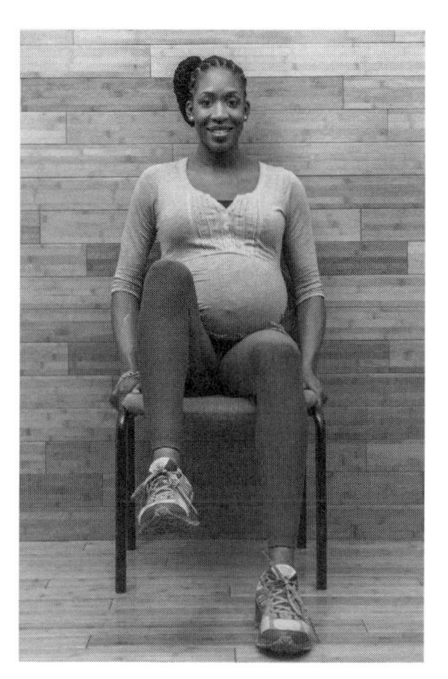
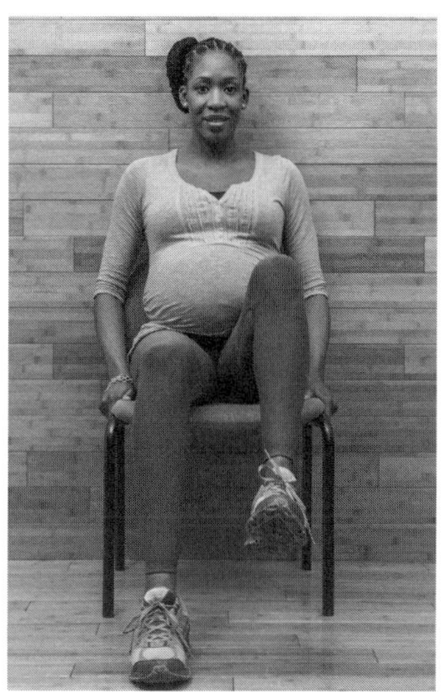
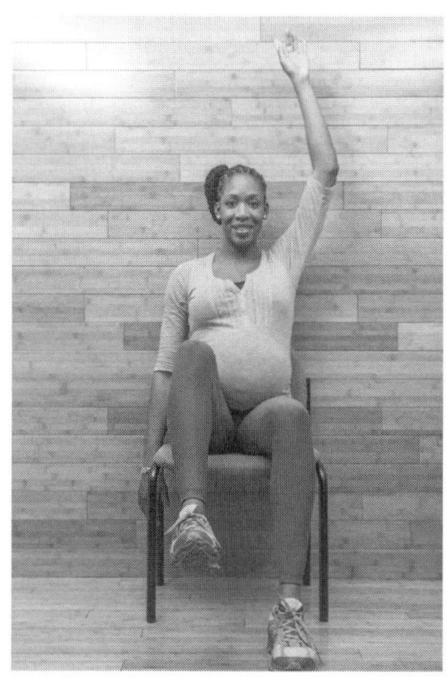
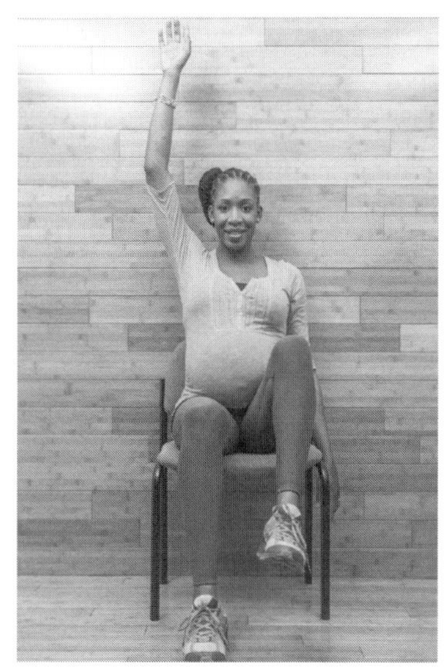

Abdominal muscle exercises

You can also practice these exercises while sitting on an exercise ball.

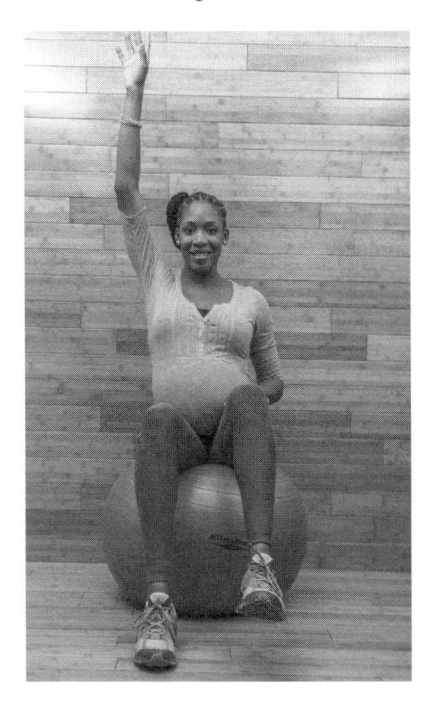

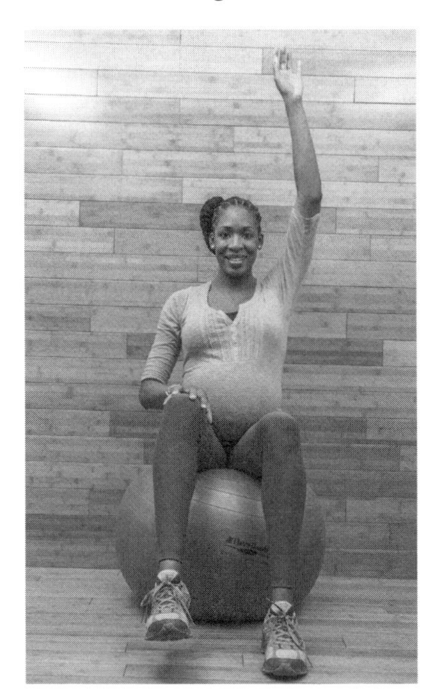

Abdominal exercises using exercise ball

You can also hold something in your hands and rotate your trunk side to side while contracting your transverse abdominal muscles.

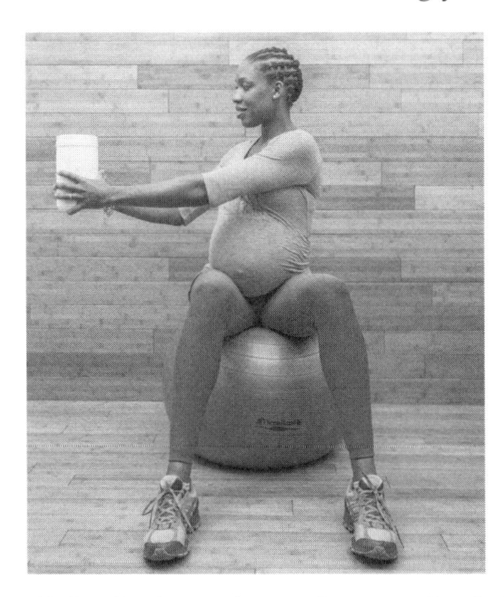

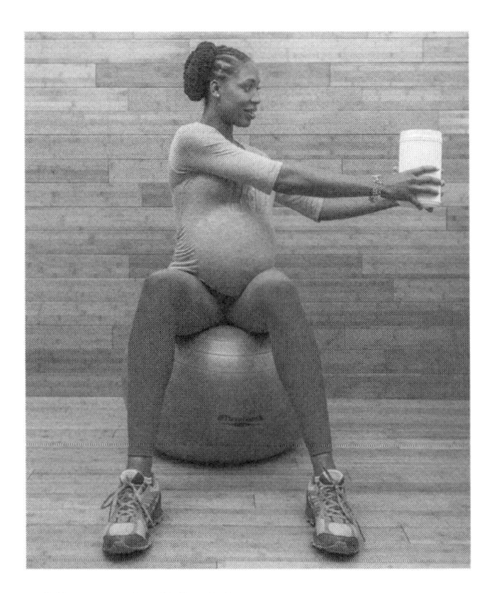

Abdominal exercises using exercise ball and household object

If you want to challenge yourself a little more, then try this:

- Place a pillow on the ground and kneel with both knees on top of it.

- Lift your feet off the floor.
- You will need to contract your transverse abdominal muscles to stay upright on your knees.

You can also do this by kneeling on your bed.

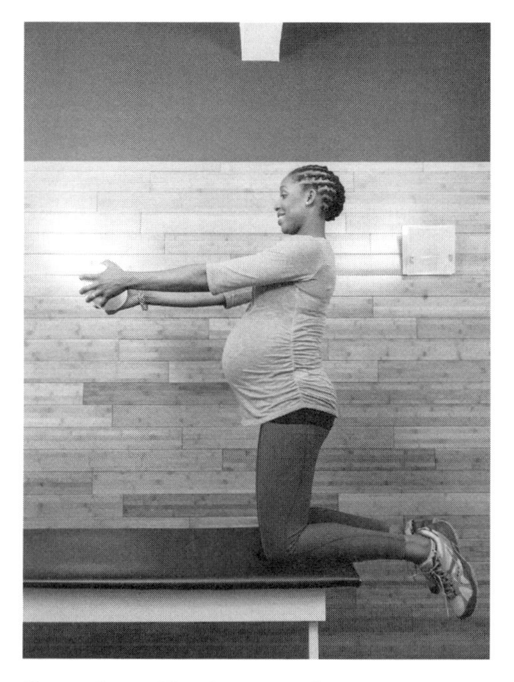

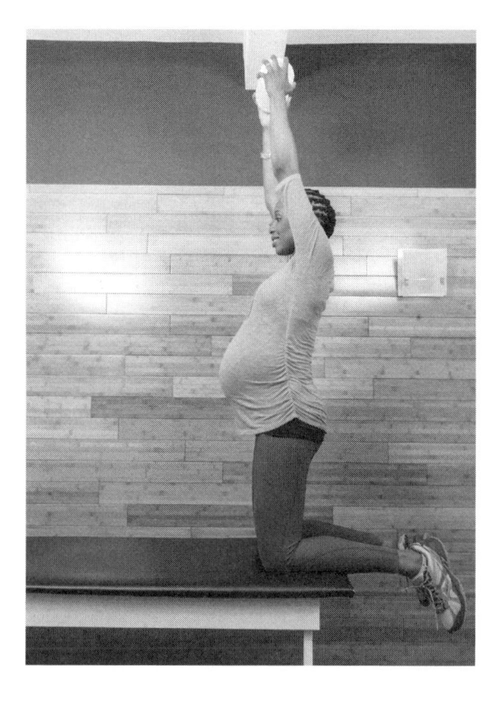

Core strengthening exercises

Here's another exercise using your handbag.

- Grab your favorite handbag (preferably with some weight to it).
- Practice pulling your belly button in toward your spine.
- Slowly raise your handbag over your head and then lower it.
- Keep your balance, keep contracting your abdominal muscles, and keep breathing!
- Now bring your handbag in front of you, chest level, with your elbows straight. Rotate the handbag to your right side, without bending your elbows. Now rotate to your left, without bending your elbows.
- Repeat each movement 10 times. This will be tough since you are working so hard to keep your balance and keeping your stomach muscles tight.

Get out of bed correctly

To prevent developing a diastasis recti:

DON'T do this:

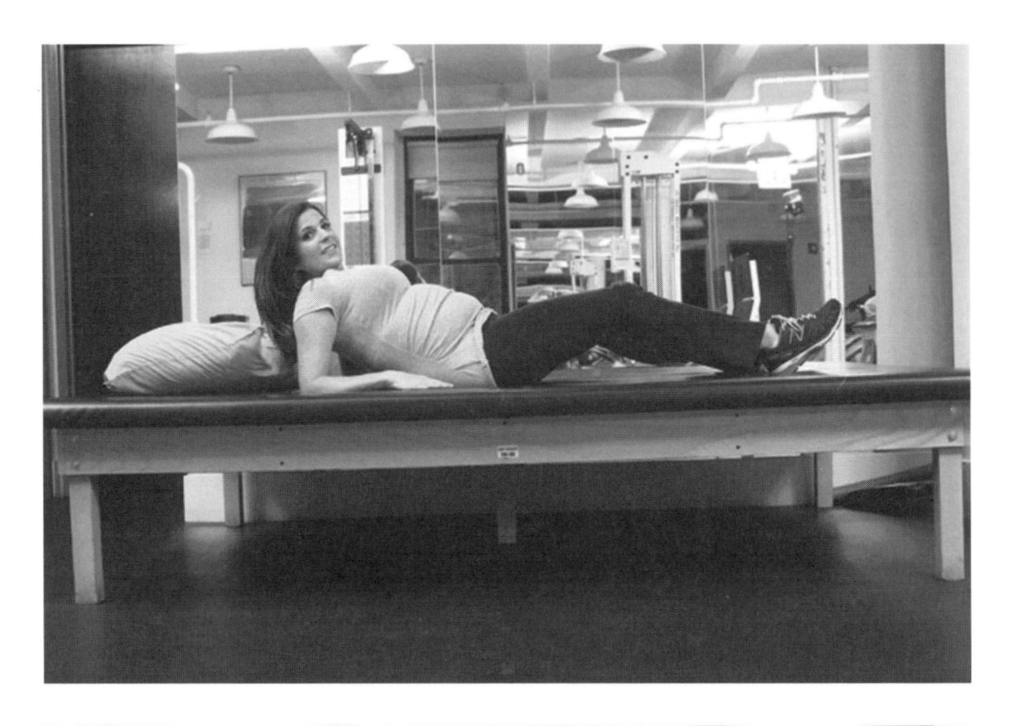

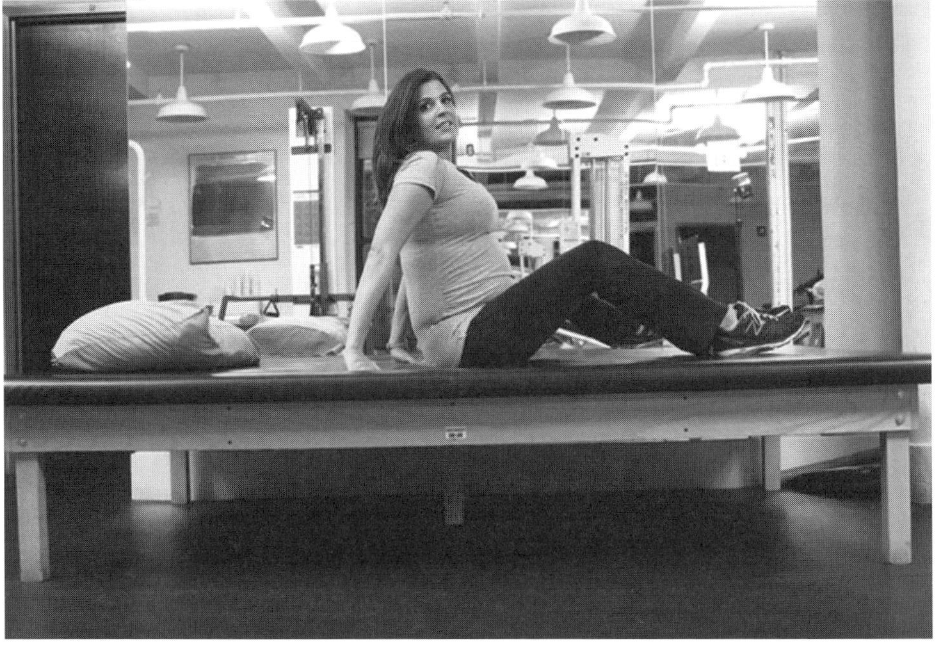

Incorrect way of getting out of bed

DO this:

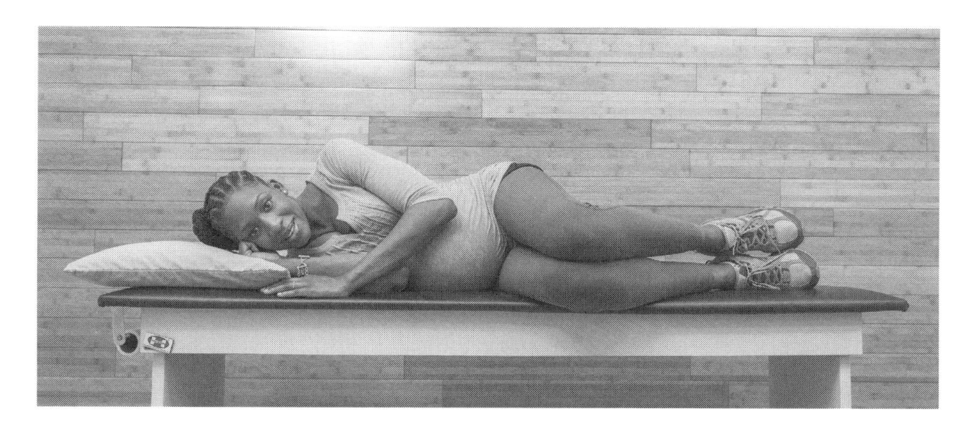

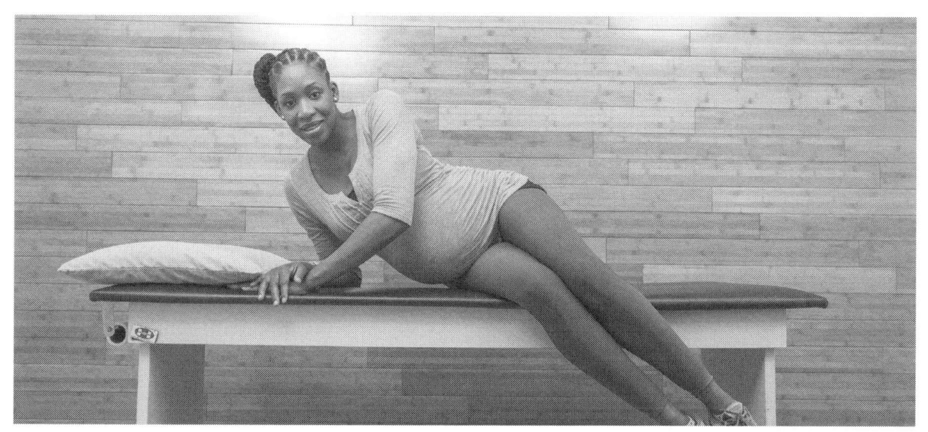

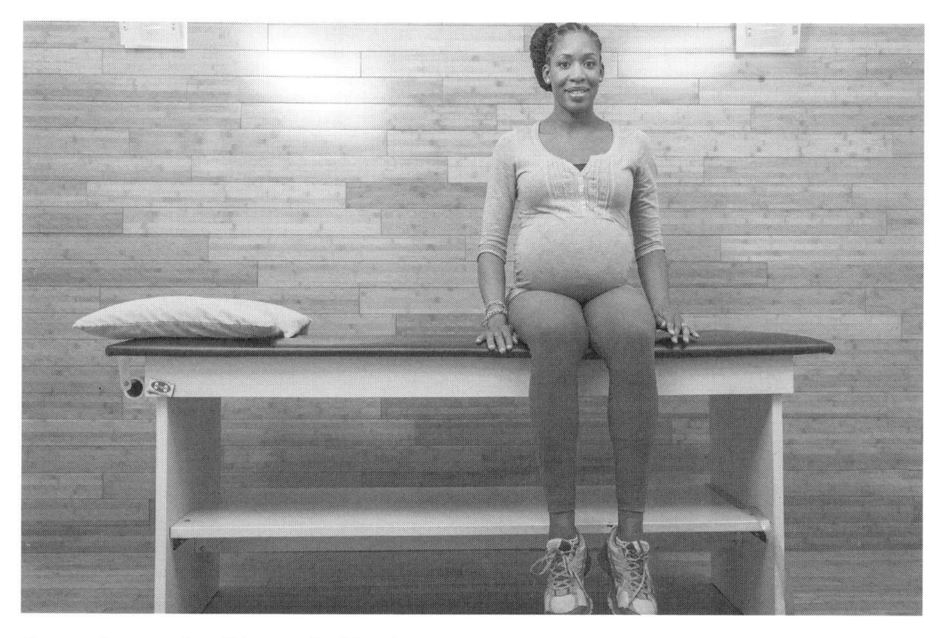

Correct way of getting out of bed

The Tupler Technique

Julie Tupler, RN, founder of the Tupler Technique®, emphasizes the importance of healing your connective tissue between your right and left abdominal muscles during your pregnancy. You want to keep it strong to prevent a diastasis from occurring if you don't have one, and preventing it from getting larger if you do have one. According to Tupler, here are three things to remember:

1. You want to correctly "position" the connective tissue to take the stretch off it versus letting it get overstretched during pregnancy. You can do this by wearing a splint to keep the muscles and connective tissue together. We don't advise this during your first trimester, when many women are nauseous. While bringing your muscles together is ideal, this will push your organs back into place and may exacerbate your nausea. Many patients enjoy wearing the splint, as it gives them more core support and helps their posture.
2. You want to protect the connective tissue from three things that weaken it:
   - Intra-abdominal force
   - Pressure
   - Stretching

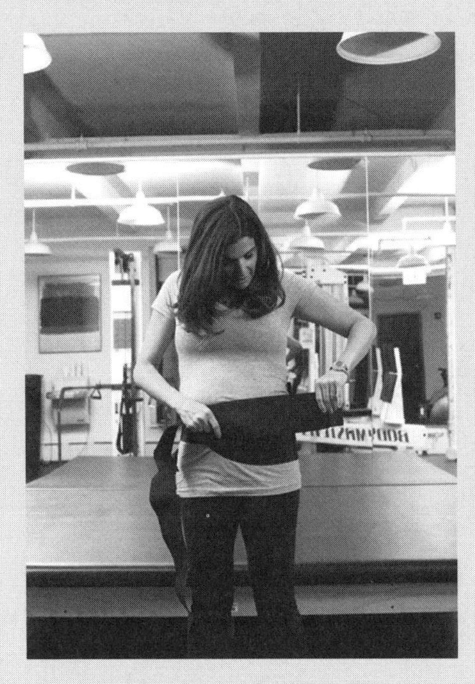

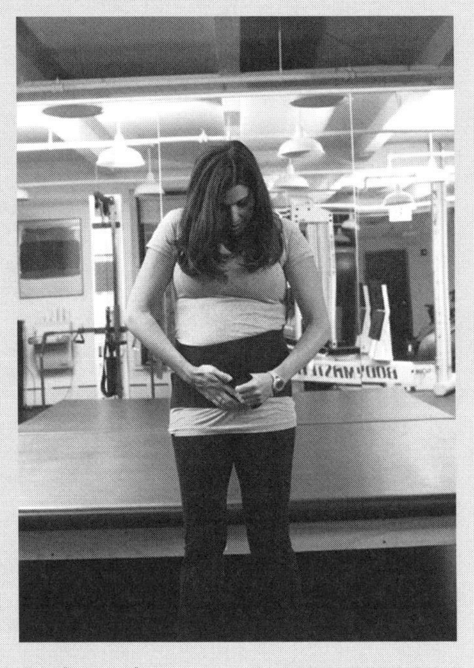

Applying the Tupler Splint to manage a diastasis recti

Intra-abdominal force on the connective tissue comes from not engaging your abdominal muscles before you move. Other examples of putting too much force on the connective tissue occur when you cough, laugh, sneeze, exercise, carry groceries, or exert yourself in any way. Huh? Try placing your hand on your belly and cough. Do you feel it come out? Now pull your belly button back toward your spine and cough again. It shouldn't move as much when you engage your transverse abdominis. Engaging these muscles protects the connective tissue and prevents a diastasis from getting larger if you have one. If you don't have one it may help prevent you from getting one.

Pressure on the connective tissue comes when you wear a front-loading baby carrier or when you exercise in a hands and knees position. In the hands and knees position, all the weight of the organs via gravity puts pressure on the connective tissue.

Stretching of the connective tissue comes from forward cross-over movements (tennis, golf) and movements that arch your upper back.

3. You want to strengthen your transverse abdominal muscles throughout the day. Strong abdominal muscles prevent back problems during and after pregnancy and help you push more effectively in labor. It is easy to get disconnected from these muscles while you're pregnant. Your belly takes over, your posture changes, and the muscles are hard to feel. Your abdominal muscles must be strong to be able to engage them during your activities of daily living and when you exercise. Remember, using your abdominal muscles prevents intra-abdominal force on your connective tissue. The harder you work to recruit and strengthen them, the easier it is to keep your diastasis as small as possible.

Our patients with back pain during their pregnancies often feel better as they strengthen these transverse abdominis muscles. Whether you opt for a natural delivery or epidural, you'll benefit from having strong abdominals to push out your baby. And if you have a C-section, you will benefit from your strong abdominals and correct body mechanics while you're recovering. We frequently hear back from our patients after having their babies. They tell us their strong abs got them through a fast(er) delivery. That's what we like to hear! As always, please consult with your midwife or doctor before starting any exercise program.

Giovanna's obstetrician cleared her to wear an abdominal splint that held her separated muscles together. She felt more supported with the splint and her nighttime back pain improved. She stopped doing core strengthening on her hands and knees and instead did transverse abdominis strengthening while sitting or kneeling. This allowed the weakened connective tissue to heal. She learned to engage her transverse abdominis muscles correctly throughout the day, especially while taking care of her other three children. This improved her posture and she stopped sticking out her stomach unintentionally. As her pregnancy progressed, she stopped complaining about her baguette. She downgraded it to a bagel stick.

Shortness of Breath

Christianna lived in a five-story apartment building in New York City without an elevator. She walked up and down four flights of steps more than once a day. After her sixth month of pregnancy, Christianna was huffing and puffing on a daily basis. She needed to take two to three rest breaks while climbing the stairs with groceries, dry cleaning, and her purse. She was spent after her daily 66-step challenge. Christianna had run several marathons in the past and didn't understand why she was having such a hard time breathing.

There are many reasons you may feel winded during your pregnancy. Feeling short of breath usually starts in the first or second trimester and is reported by 75 percent of healthy pregnant women by their 30th week. It is common to feel like you just can't take a deep breath. Your breaths are short and fast. Your progesterone hormone is partially to blame here. In addition to causing constipation and reflux, it stimulates respiration. This makes you feel like you are breathing quickly. These changes may make it hard for your lungs to fully expand. This may cause more shallow breathing, and you may feel short of breath.

It isn't surprising that your uterus pushes other abdominal organs out of the way as it grows. It pushes up on the diaphragm around the 31st to 34th week. The diaphragm is an abdominal muscle under your rib cage and is a key muscle in helping you breathe. When your diaphragm isn't functioning at full capacity, your lungs can't fully expand and your breathing becomes more shallow. But don't worry! Eventually the baby will drop and your diaphragm will have a little more room to move. Let's learn a little more about how your diaphragm works.

Your diaphragm is a dome- or parachute-shaped muscle sitting tucked up under your ribs. This muscle moves with every breath that you take. Every time you breathe in, the diaphragm moves downward toward your abdomen. During each exhale, your diaphragm moves up and pushes the air in your lungs out. This is something that you don't need to think about since it is an automatic function in your body. You can imagine how the presence of a little bundle in your abdomen might block the diaphragm from doing what it normally does.

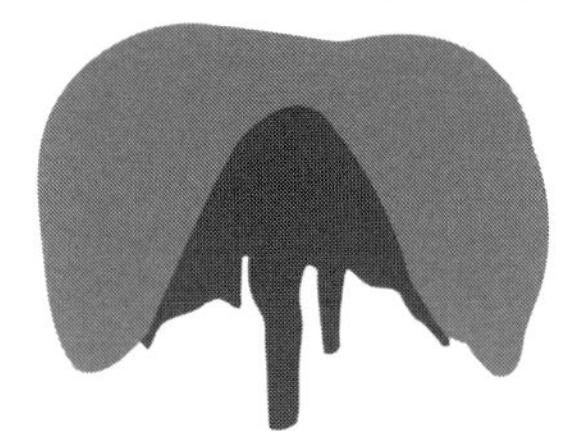

The diaphragm is shaped like a parachute

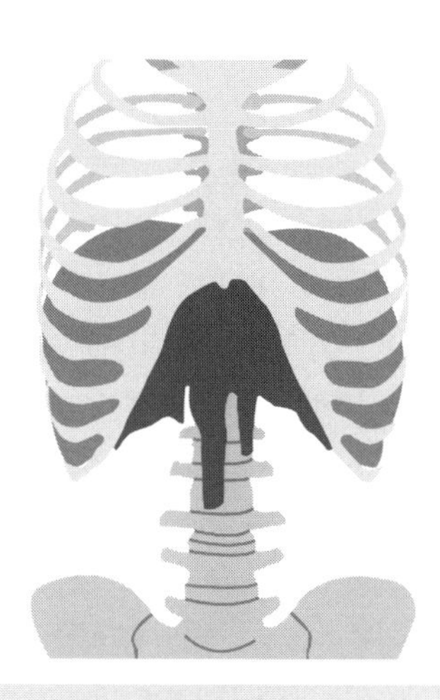

Yes, You Do Have a Big Head

I'm sure sometime in your life, someone has accused you of having a "big head." Is that an insult? No! It's a fact. You do, indeed, have a big head. Everyone does. And it's quite heavy as well. The average adult human head weighs between 8 and 12 pounds. That's a lot to hold up! Your muscles are working hard to support the weight of your head and control head movement. These muscles are your postural muscles. Every second that you are upright, these postural muscles are at work. They also function as your *secondary* respiratory muscles. These *secondary* respiratory muscles need to focus on the *primary* job of holding up your head. They can't be bothered with your breathing. The muscle that really needs to be focusing on your breathing is your diaphragm.

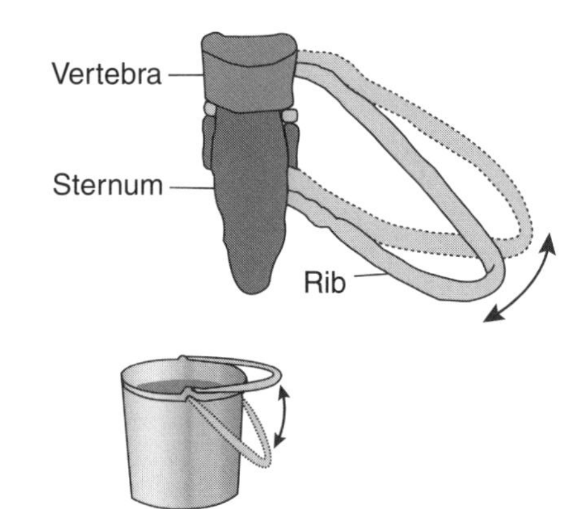

Another motion that occurs during respiration is the movement of your ribs. Your ribs need to move out in order for your diaphragm to allow air into your lungs. This movement is almost like a bucket handle. As you breathe in, your bucket handle (ribs) move up and out. As you breathe out, the bucket handle returns to its resting position.

What you can do

So let's talk about ways that you can improve your respiration. Remember, your baby needs the oxygen too.

Diaphragmatic breathing

This is an ideal exercise to start early on in the pregnancy before you even start to show. Your breathing pattern will change as your baby grows. Starting the pregnancy with a proper and efficient breathing pattern is important for you and your baby.

Let's begin this exercise leaning back in a chair.

Place both your hands on your belly, or one hand on your chest and the other on your belly. Try to become as relaxed as you possibly can. Clear your mind of your mile-long to-do list, possible baby name list, and "things I need to add to my registry" list. Focus on *how* you are breathing. Are you using more of your upper chest muscles? Are you taking short and shallow breaths? Or are you taking long, slow, deep breaths? Are you able to count to five while you inhale and while you exhale? Try your best to keep your upper hand "quiet."

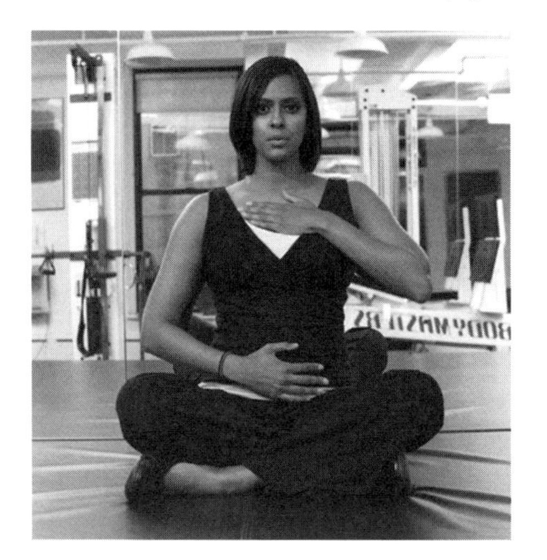

Diaphragmatic breathing

Move your bottom hand *outward* when you breathe *in*. Let your bottom hand come back toward your spine when you breathe out.

Relax your shoulders and your chest. Most people hold their tension here, so try and release all your tension.

Try to have the movement of your breathing come from your abdomen. Visualize your breath entering through your nose and heading down into your abdomen. As the breath passes through your body, it zaps all the tension and leaves behind loose, relaxed muscles. Feel your abdomen fill with air. As you exhale, let the air out through your mouth slowly.

Sleeping Beauty

You breathe properly when you sleep. You are not tense when you sleep (unless you are having a nightmare about the awful shade of green that your partner picked for the nursery). You diaphragmatically breathe when you are sleeping. So try to get as relaxed as you can without falling asleep and you'll see your breathing pattern change. Try to be aware of how this feels and see how much of it you can control. See if you can bring on this natural breathing pattern at least once a day. Make the time to be relaxed and work that primary muscle of respiration, the diaphragm.

Babies also breathe properly. They use their diaphragms and breathe efficiently. They haven't learned yet to be stressed out and use their secondary respiratory muscles instead of their diaphragm. Maybe you have another little one running around the house from whom you can get tips on how to breathe.

Strengthening your intercostal muscles

As your pregnancy progresses, your baby will be taking up more and more space in your belly. This will prevent your diaphragm from going through its full range of motion. You can still practice deep breathing throughout your pregnancy but now we are going to work on strengthening the muscles between your ribs (your intercostal muscles) to help you expand your ribs/lungs more and take a deeper breath. Here's a way you can strengthen these respiratory muscles, make your breathing efficient, and get your ribs moving.

- Wrap a resistance band around your back, keeping it level around your lower ribs. (Remember, your diaphragm is tucked under these lower ribs). Criss cross the resistance band and add tension by pulling on the ends. Keep that tension at all times.
- Now take those long, slow, deep breaths against the resistance of the bands. Remember to keep your upper chest quiet. You can also have your partner put his or her hands over your low ribs. Practice breathing into your partner's hands. They can also apply slight resistance in order to help strengthen the muscles between your ribs.

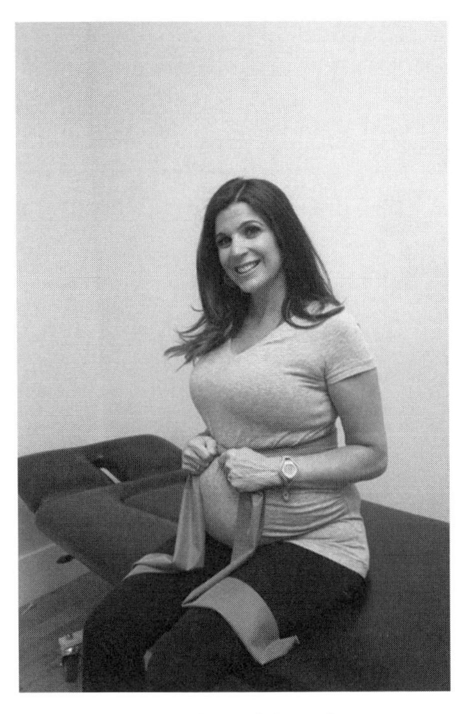

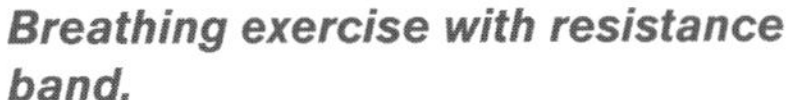

Breathing exercise with resistance band.

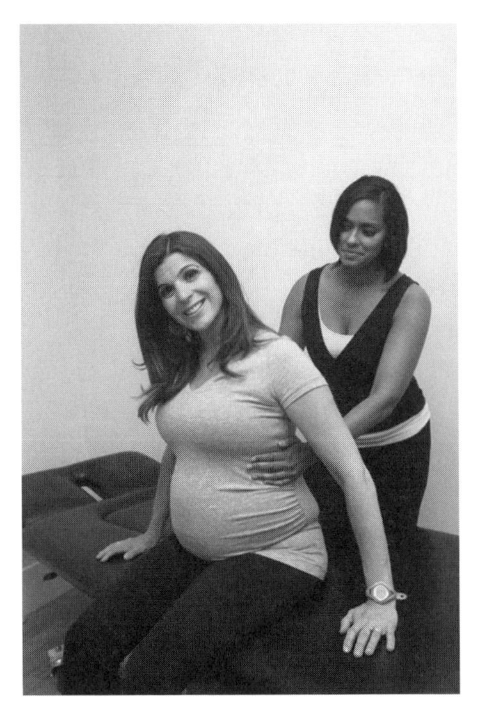

Breathing exercise with partner.

Don't hold your breath at any point, and stop if you feel fatigued.

Try doing a set of 10 and breathe through a count of five seconds. (You'll also be giving your arms a workout.) Take breaks as you need them and try doing another set of 10 when you are ready.

Keep building up your breathing endurance. Your breathing muscles are just like any other muscles—they need to be worked out. It's important to incorporate these muscles and your breathing exercises into your exercise program.

Stretch your intercostal muscles

You also can stretch these intercostal muscles that are between your ribs. Sometimes these muscles can become tight, especially if you hold a lot of tension in your upper body.

You can try this stretch sitting in a chair or half kneeling on the floor.

- Simply reach one hand overhead and lean to the opposite side. Reach over until you feel a stretch on your side. This stretch is good for the muscles between your ribs as well as the muscles along the side of your trunk.
- Hold each stretch for 30 seconds. And don't forget to breathe deeply!

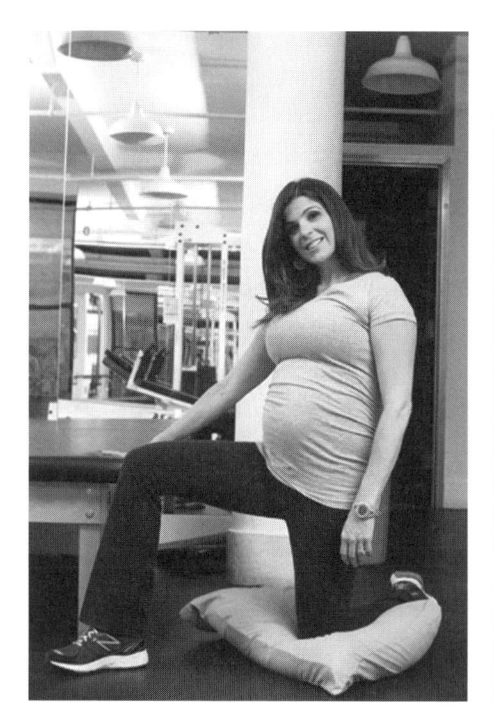
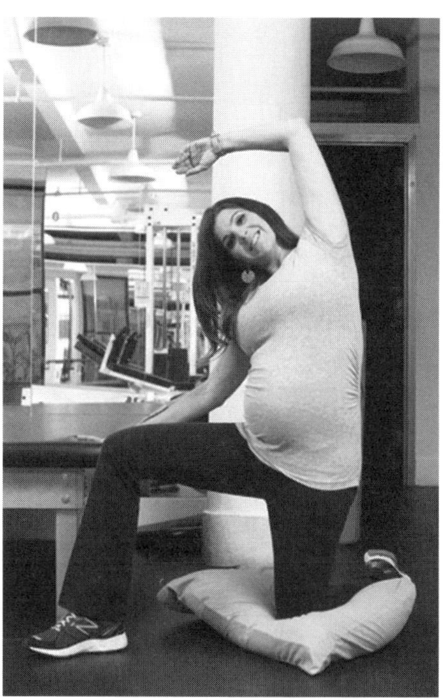

Side trunk/rib stretch

Christianna practiced breathing against a resistance band daily as described. While she still needed to take a break at the third floor landing and found herself panting once she made it to her apartment, she reported a notable difference. The 66 steps were still challenging, but her daily activities were much easier.

Sleeping Pains

Lori noticed that her bed was getting more and more crowded every night. There was Lori, lots of pillows, her growing belly, oh, and that's right, her partner. Lori wanted to know how she could support her belly, cuddle with her partner, and sleep comfortably without falling off the bed due to all these new components in her bedroom.

Having the right position and proper support from pillows is an important factor for getting a good night's rest. We let Lori know that falling asleep on her left side is the safest position. As her baby grows, the growing uterus will put increasing pressure on important blood vessels, the inferior vena cava and aorta. These are the largest artery and vein in your body. Compression of these vessels in the abdomen can impede blood flow to the heart and legs. When the pressure is too much, women will literally receive a wake-up call. They may begin to sweat; notice a change in their pulses; or feel dizzy, nauseous, or lightheaded. These conditions affect 10 percent to 20 percent of women during their pregnancies.

What you can do

Lie on your left side or on your back with your right hip propped up at least 15 degrees with a wedge or pillow. The good news is, most pregnant women are inclined to tilt to their left sides while sleeping in their third trimester. Researchers looked at sleep positions of pregnant and non-pregnant women and there was a significant difference. The majority of the pregnant group adopted a sleeping position that reduced the likelihood of aortocaval compression syndrome.

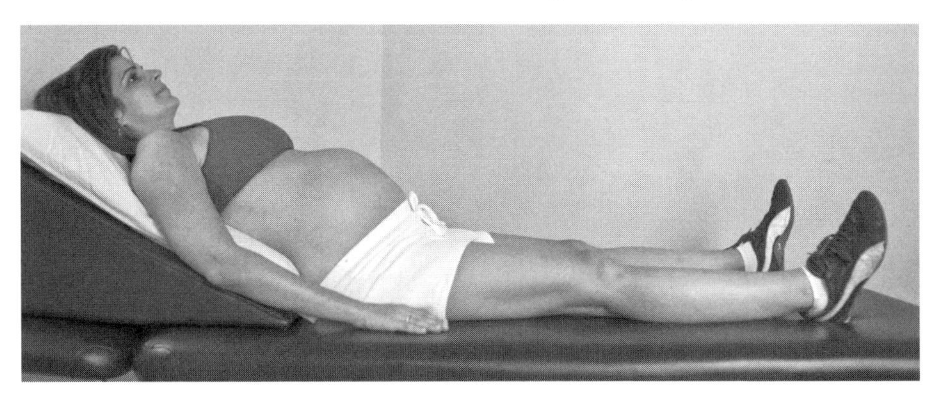

Safe positioning with pillow to prevent compression of blood vessels while lying on back

So how should you sleep? Use a pillow under your top leg to keep your pelvis aligned and hips in a neutral position. Pregnant or not, side sleepers should use a pillow. Without it, your top hip rotates inward and puts unnecessary strain on your hip and low back. Using a pillow behind your back will help provide extra support and prevent you from rolling back. And since you are already on a pillow-stealing binge, why not take one more? Some women feel better with a pillow under their bellies while they're lying on their left side. This relieves some pulling and strain at the low back. A body pillow will be helpful at this point. As your pregnancy progresses, you may need to say farewell to your partner, as there may not be enough room for all of you!

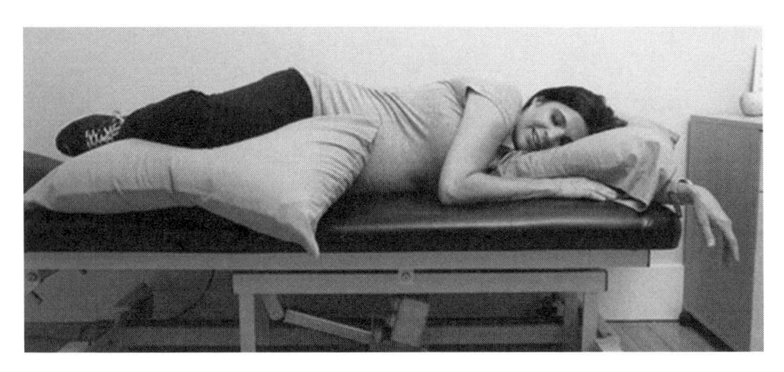

Sleeping position using pillows

Are You a Belly Sleeper?

If you are a belly sleeper, you are probably missing your favorite sleeping position as you grow bigger. Don't fret! There are several options available for sleeping pillows that allow pregnant women to sleep on their tummies. These cushions have spaces or cutouts for the pregnant belly and sometimes for the pregnant boobs. These pillows are fairly expensive. Our patients have fabricated their own versions with pillows and an inflatable swimming tube.

Got GERD?

You just ate a bucket of Buffalo wings and are wondering why that burning sensation in your chest won't go away. Don't worry, it might have been there even if you only had one wing. According to a study done by the College of Family Physicians of Canada, gastroesophageal reflux disease (GERD) is reported in up to 80 percent of pregnancies. It is most likely caused by an increase in progesterone. Progesterone, designed to relax the smooth muscles in your uterus, also relaxes the valve that separates the esophagus from the stomach. Hormonal changes in pregnancy can also decrease movement in the gastrointestinal tract, which results in slower digestion and an increased risk of reflux. Also, as your baby continues to grow, your little bundle occupies more and more of the space in your tummy. This causes more and more stomach acids to be pushed back up the esophagus, which causes that unpleasant burning sensation.

The easiest thing you can do to relieve some of these symptoms of heartburn and reflux is to make some lifestyle changes. You can try eating smaller and more frequent meals. And make sure you eat that last small meal way before bedtime. Also, you can try sleeping on a wedge (or several pillows) so that your upper body is slightly propped up, which may relieve some of the symptoms of reflux. Additionally:

- Eat slowly.
- Drink fluids between meals—not with meals.
- Don't eat greasy and fried foods.
- Avoid citrus fruits or juices and spicy foods.
- Do not eat or drink within a few hours of bedtime.
- Do not lie down right after meals.

Swelling

Jenifer was worried about her swollen ankles. Her socks were cutting off the circulation in her legs and she was worried about a blood clot after doing some Internet research. Her swelling would worsen throughout the day and, by the evenings, she could barely stand anymore. She was six months' pregnant and had a two-year-old to take care of, so lying down with her legs elevated wasn't an option for her.

Do You Also Have Cankles?

During pregnancy, you have extra blood volume throughout your body. Eight out of ten women have clinical edema (swelling) at some point during their pregnancy. You are carrying around an additional six to eight liters of water. No wonder you feel like a two gallon water balloon.

The swelling may seem worse in your feet and ankles because your growing uterus puts pressure on the blood vessels in your pelvis. Your inferior vena cava is the largest vein in your body and carries blood from your legs back to your heart. When it is compressed by your growing uterus, the blood flow slows down and pools in your legs.

Swelling is often worst in the third trimester and at the end of the day. Humidity and flying will worsen your sausage-like legs, so a trip to the Caribbean rain forest is not an ideal babymoon destination. While some swelling in the feet and ankles is considered normal during pregnancy, your doctor should be notified if it is severe. If you can press your thumb into your lower leg and still see a thumbprint after you pull your hand away, you may have pitting edema. If you notice swelling in your face or puffiness around your eyes, contact your doctor or midwife immediately. These could be symptoms of preeclampsia, high

Fun Fact: Your Baby's Hair Actually Might Cause Your Heartburn

A study performed at Johns Hopkins Medical Institution showed that there does in fact appear to be an association between heartburn severity during pregnancy and newborn hair. It is believed there is a shared biologic mechanism involving a dual role of pregnancy hormones in both the relaxation of the lower esophageal sphincter and the modulation of fetal hair growth.

blood pressure, and excess protein in the urine that if left untreated can lead to serious—even fatal—complications for both you and your baby.

How Do You Know If You Have Preeclampsia?

According to the University of Maryland Medical Center, you may not even experience symptoms if you have mild preeclampsia. During each prenatal visit, however, your health care provider will measure your blood pressure, test your urine, and be on the lookout for other early signs of the disease—a good reason not to miss any of your checkups.

Symptoms include:

- Blood pressure of 140/90 or higher on two separate occasions at least six hours apart
- Protein in your urine
- Swelling in the hands and face

Symptoms of **severe** preeclampsia include:

- Blurred vision or spots in front of your eyes
- Sensitivity to light
- Lethargy
- Nausea and vomiting
- Severe swelling
- Sudden weight gain of more than a pound a day
- Shortness of breath
- Exaggerated reflexes
- A headache that does not go away
- Belly pain below the ribs on the right side
- Right shoulder pain
- Decreased urine output
- Irritability

Your doctor will perform a physical exam and run some tests before making this diagnosis. The treatment is to deliver the baby! If it is too early in your pregnancy, you may be placed on bed rest either at home or in the hospital. Symptoms usually subside within six weeks of delivering, but your blood pressure may worsen within the first few days. And, unlucky you … if you have preeclampsia once, you are more likely to develop it again in another pregnancy. However, it is not usually as severe as the first time.

The cause of preeclampsia is unknown, but if this is your first pregnancy or you're carrying multiples, you are at risk. If you're over 35, have a history of diabetes, and are obese, you've hit all the risk factors.

For more information on preeclampsia, visit: preeclampsia.org.

What you can do

It's good to know the swelling will resolve after delivery, but what can you do for it now?

- **Stay hydrated.** The Institute of Medicine recommends about 10 cups (2.3 liters) of fluids a day during pregnancy. We know it may seem counter-intuitive to drink more water while you're already retaining too much, but it will help. Proper hydration improves your circulation so you won't accumulate excessive pooling in your legs. Plus, more trips to the bathroom mean you won't be sitting or standing for too long, which leads us to the next tip.
- **Sleep on your left side if you can**. This takes pressure off the inferior vena cava so there will be less blood flow restriction.
- **Discuss the option of maternity compression stockings or socks with your doctor or midwife.** The additional support will improve the circulation in your legs, resulting in decreased swelling. The lowest level starts at 8 to 15 mmHg and gets as high as 50–60 mmHg. Don't be surprised by the price of these. They're expensive, but your legs will thank you.
- **Elevate your legs above your heart as much as possible while sitting or lying down.** You have a good reason to steal all the pillows. You can even raise the foot of your bed to elevate your swollen limbs while sleeping.
- **Exercise.** Take a power walk outside or exercise indoors at the gym or your home. Cool down in the pool and swim some laps. Exercising your leg muscles will help your circulation and move the fluid out of your legs.

Please know, if one leg is significantly more swollen than the other, you should contact your doctor or midwife. This may be the result of a vascular condition, arthritis, lymphedema, blood clot, gout, infection, tumor, or other condition that requires medical attention. Please don't ignore your swollen limb.

How Much Salt Can I Have?

Please note, we did not recommend that you decrease the sodium in your diet (assuming you currently consume a moderate amount in your diet). This is a controversial topic and the medical recommendations have shifted. Doctors used to tell women to decrease their sodium levels to lower their blood pressure and decrease water retention. No pickles for them! In 2011, German researchers conducted an animal study to study the effects of sodium in the pregnant females. It was concluded that both excessively high and excessively low levels of sodium during pregnancy have an adverse effect on kidney development in the offspring.

So how much salt should you consume? The World Health Organization recommends less than 2,000 milligrams of sodium a day (¾ to 1 teaspoon of salt) and the American Heart Association recommends limiting sodium to less than 1,500 milligrams a day (½ to ¾ teaspoon of salt). Americans average 3,600 milligrams per day, doubling the recommended consumption, according to the American Heart Association. These guidelines don't change during pregnancy. So you can have that pickle you are craving … just cut it in half.

Jenifer stopped self-diagnosing and assuming the worst from what she read online. While she hated the idea of maternity support hose, she purchased some and they helped her immensely. She modified her work and exercise schedule too. She didn't have the option of elevating her swollen legs in her small work cubicle, so she took frequent breaks to walk around her office, which improved her blood circulation. She walked for four to five minutes every hour. While she initially told us she was too busy to take breaks, she got hooked on the practice. She interacted with colleagues she normally didn't see, had less leg discomfort and swelling, and felt better mentally when she took breaks from the monotony of typing. When the weather permitted, she started walking with a friend for 30 minutes after work. This improved her swollen legs and energy level in the evening.

Tailbone Pain (Coccyx Pain)

Kris was unable to sit during her third trimester due to tailbone pain. She developed low back pain from standing all day, as this was the only position she could tolerate. Her obstetrician referred her to an orthopedic doctor, who said he couldn't help her because she was pregnant. She was told she would feel better after delivering her baby, who was putting too much pressure on her tailbone.

At this point, you've been sitting in your doctor or midwife's waiting room for hours and you think that this is a pain in the ass. Or you may actually have a pain in the ass. Your tailbone, also known as your coccyx, is a little bone connected to the base of your spine. Your tailbone needs to move in order for you to deliver your baby (and to poop!). Just like all your other joints, this little joint is also being affected by your pregnancy hormones. The tailbone can feel tender and maybe even move a little too much during your pregnancy. It can be extremely uncomfortable to sit for a long time or get up from a chair.

What you can do

Since you can't put off your gestational diabetes test forever, when you finally go to the lab, bring a cushion with you. You will be glad you have it as you wait for your bloodwork to be completed. And while you pray that the test is negative so you don't have to give up donuts, donut cushions are *not* the answer. Donut cushions are good for other pelvic conditions such as trauma to your perineum after delivery, but *not* for sacroiliac pain or tailbone pain. These cushions actually make the condition worse because they are compressing the areas that are actually causing you pain.

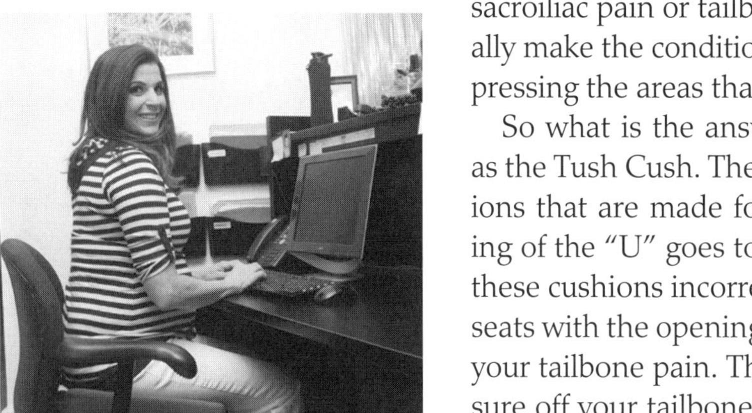

Using a seating cushion at the workstation for proper posture and comfort

So what is the answer? U-shaped cushions, such as the Tush Cush. There are wedged U-shaped cushions that are made for this type of pain. The opening of the "U" goes to the *back*. People generally use these cushions incorrectly, and sit on them like toilet seats with the opening in the front. This won't relieve your tailbone pain. The wedge shape takes the pressure off your tailbone by tipping your pelvis forward and restoring your low back curvature. So take this with you on long drives, to doctor appointments, your office, or restaurants. Take it wherever you will be sitting for long periods of time and you'll notice a definite decrease in your tailbone pain.

Kris's preg head made her forget where she put her Tush Cush one too many times. She kept leaving it places and got tired of replacing it. She did feel better when she used it and was happy to finally sit without pain. She corrected her standing posture and was able to relax her pelvic floor muscles. This was significant for two reasons—it reduced the pressure on her tailbone and helped get her pelvis ready for labor.

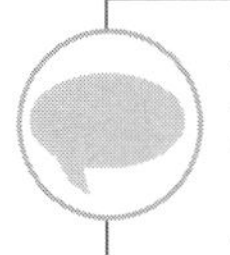

From Denise: I am a triathlete and spend a lot of time sitting on a bike. Sometimes it's a spin bike at the gym, but most of the time it's my road bike. Sitting on a small bike seat for hours definitely causes its fair share of bum pain—even while wearing a pair of bike shorts with butt padding that makes it look like I am wearing a diaper. Whenever I have pain in my bum from riding, I use this cushion for long car rides or sitting at my desk. I'm also diligent about performing the stretches and strengthening exercises that we mention in the pelvic pain section of this chapter (page 42). So don't worry if you have a pain in the ass. Be dedicated about taking care of it and it will feel better.

Learning to relax your pelvic floor muscles is also an important part of easing tailbone pain. There are muscles in your pelvis that connect directly to your tailbone. If the muscles are tight, then that can cause tailbone pain. There are several things you can do to relax your pelvic floor muscles. In the section on pelvic pain in this chapter (page 42), we review stretches you can do to target the tight muscles in your pelvis.

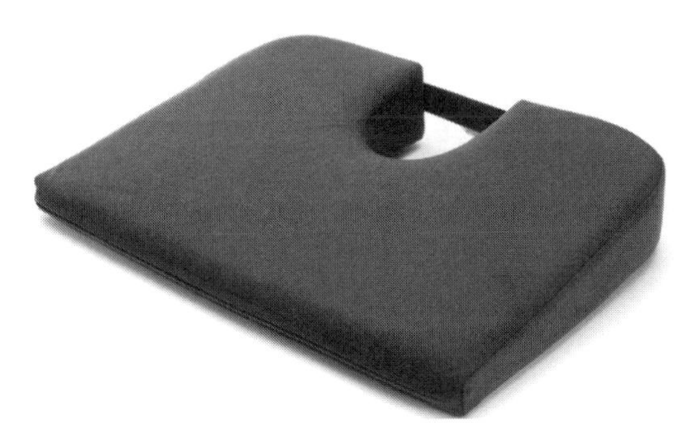

The Tush Cush

Varicose Veins

Brenda stayed active throughout her pregnancy. She taught martial arts and ran three times a week. Her swollen and bluish legs scared her running partner and class participants more than her medical team. Her socks left indentations in her swollen calves. Her skin looked like it was going to burst open. She felt best after exercising. Her doctors said the varicosities would resolve after delivery, like they did after her previous two pregnancies, so they weren't concerned. Her biggest problem was sleeping at night. Her legs throbbed and kept her awake. She had dull pain in her lower abdomen and she developed varicose veins around her vagina. She was afraid to have sex and didn't know how she would deliver a baby without rupturing her inflamed veins.

Don't let these blue veins make you blue. Varicose veins are superficial, twisted, and enlarged veins most commonly seen in the legs. Healthy veins have one-way valves that help keep the blood flowing back to your heart. If the valves get weakened or damaged, the deoxygenated blood pools in your legs. This increased pressure can cause pain, fatigue, achiness, heaviness, burning, or throbbing for some women. Others don't experience any pain, but have swelling and skin discoloration. And yet some women report no symptoms.

Varicose veins are a common condition during pregnancy, seen in 33 percent of women after delivering their first baby and 55 percent in women who have delivered two or more babies, not including twins. The great saphenous vein, found in the inside of your leg, is a common area to have varicosities. (You can often see and feel this vein on your inner knee.)

What are the risk factors?

- Women are two to three times more likely than men to develop varicose veins
- Obesity or excessive weight gain
- Family history
- Age: between 30 and 70 years old
- Pregnancy
- Use of birth control pills
- Prolonged standing or sitting

From Jill: I don't mean to strive for perfection, but I give myself a perfect score here. I received my first pair of support hose as a teenager. Just what every girl wants. During my waitressing days, I was on my feet for several hours a day. Since my mom developed painful varicose veins during her two pregnancies, she was kind enough to share her stockings so I could avoid her struggles. So just like my mom, I donned my support hose to work. But unlike my mom, I wore a stained International House of Pancakes dress over them.

Why are they worse during pregnancy? Blame it on the hormones once again. Researchers have studied whether pregnancy alone can cause varicose veins or if elevated hormones are the culprits. Blood work in pregnant women with varicose veins was compared to the blood work in women without them. It was concluded that women with varicose veins had significantly higher levels of progesterone, the hormone that plays a role in maintaining pregnancy.

Additionally, the veins in your legs are enlarged from your increased blood volume and the impact of your growing uterus. Your uterus puts pressure on the veins in your pelvis, which impedes the blood flow from your legs and consequently causes increased pressure and pooling in the veins.

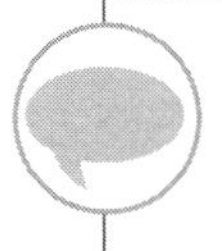

Please note ladies, crossing your legs won't give you varicose veins. This old wives' tale has been repeatedly disproven.

These swollen veins aren't isolated to your legs. You can develop them at your rectum and anus, where they are called hemorrhoids. The good news is, they often resolve after delivery. The bad news is, pushing can make them worse. For your hemorrhoids, please read our section on constipation.

Vulvar varicosities are varicose veins in the vulva. Who knew there were so many places to develop varicose veins? The vulva includes all the external female genitalia. Vulvar varicosities are generally not an indication for a cesarean section. If you are worried about tearing, having an episiotomy, or rupturing the varicosities during labor, then please discuss this with your doctor or midwife. Research, however, shows that women with vulvar varicosities can be allowed to attempt a vaginal birth regardless of their severity.

What you can do

While there is no cure for varicose veins, here are some tips for keeping your veins strong and healthy:

- Stay active to keep your muscles strong and facilitate good circulation in your legs.
- Follow your doctor's or midwife's weight gain recommendation.

- Elevate your legs above your heart when resting as much as possible.
- Sleep on the left side so your uterus doesn't put pressure on your inferior vena cava, which is the large vein carrying blood from your legs to your heart.
- Don't stand or sit for long periods of time. If standing for prolonged periods is unavoidable, shift your weight to each leg frequently. Make sure to take breaks once or twice an hour if you're sitting for extended periods.
- Wear maternity elastic support stockings. Though they have not been proven to prevent varicose veins during pregnancy, they have been shown to improve leg symptoms and prevent pooling at the groin.
- Wear vulvar support garments (or you can put a maxi pad in a pair of maternity biker shorts).
- Avoid tight clothing and belts.
- Avoid high heels. Wearing low heels or sneakers will use your leg muscles more efficiently and help your circulation.

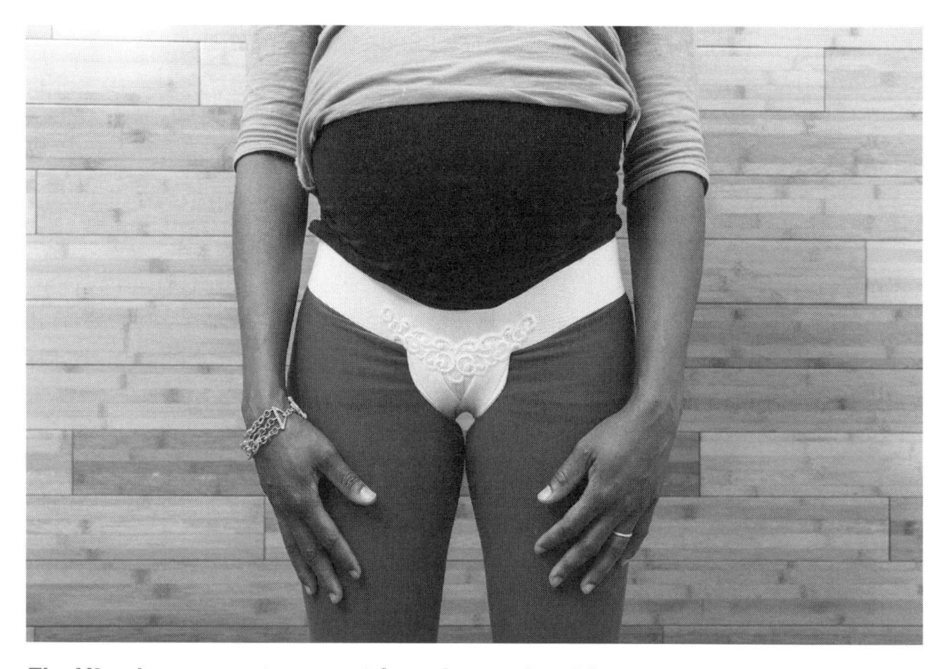

The V2 vulvar support garment for vulvar varicosities

- Maternity belts and pregnancy supports can decrease the pressure in the abdomen and pelvis to improve blood flow.

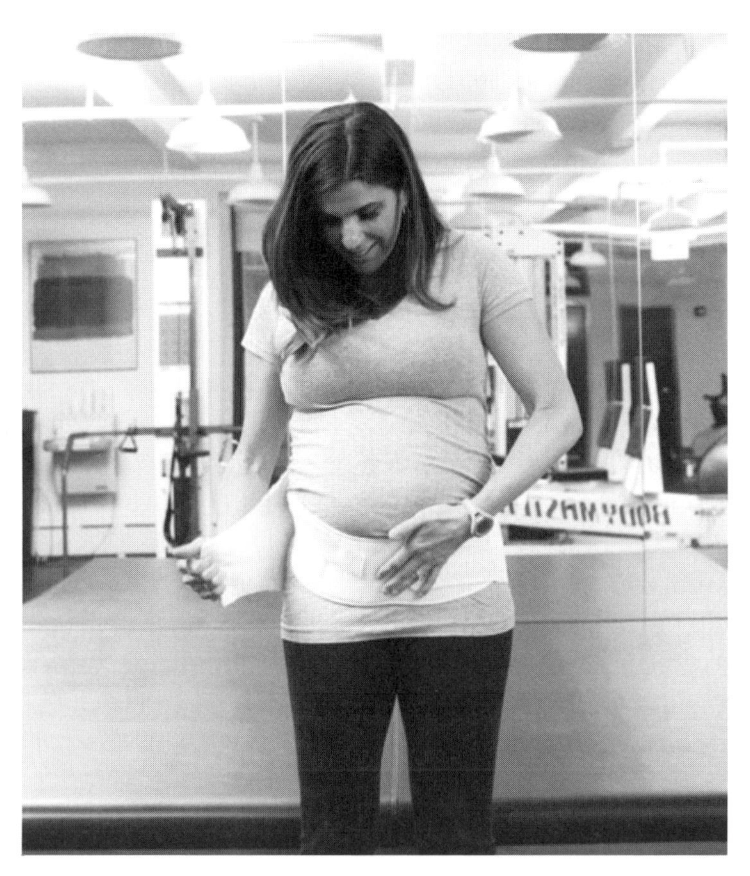

Maternal supports can lift the belly to improve leg circulation and varicose veins

Brenda's doctors were right. Her varicosities disappeared within three and a half weeks after delivery. All of them! She wore compression socks daily. She wore compression stockings in the evenings, which decreased the throbbing in her legs and allowed her to sleep. She tried a perineal support garment for her vaginal varicosities and found it too uncomfortable. She was still afraid to have sex, so she refrained until her vaginal varicosities subsided. She had a planned C-section without any complications.

Additional Help from Acupuncture and Chinese Herbal Medicine

As physical therapists, we can help alleviate many of the discomforts of pregnancy, but there are some that are outside our area of expertise.

Since we can't help you with your morning sickness, anemia, and either breeched or overdue babies, we refer to a profession that can! Acupuncture and Chinese herbal medicine have been practiced for centuries and are used for a myriad of health problems, including pregnancy symptoms. Many of our patients have experienced the benefits. We consulted with acupuncturists and Chinese Medicine Herbalists Jill Blakeway, MSc, LAC, and Mary Sabo, MSc, LAC, at the YinOva Center in New York City.

Here is what they had to share.

Acupuncture

Acupuncture is a good choice for many pregnancy ailments because it offers drug-free relief for a number of disorders. We often use it as relief for conditions that people see as a normal part of pregnancy, such as morning sickness, sciatica, back pain, pubic pain, edema, and fatigue. We also use it before the birth to promote an efficient labor or to initiate labor in women who are past their due date. We use moxa and acupuncture to help breech babies turn into a safe position for delivery.

It's important to pick an acupuncturist with experience in obstetrics because there are acupuncture points that are contraindicated in pregnancy because of their tendency to promote contractions. However, in the hands of a well-trained and qualified acupuncturist, acupuncture is an extremely safe form of treatment for pregnant women.

The following conditions are treated with acupuncture, but you can also practice them with applied pressure at home. Any point we discuss can be used for acupressure simply by applying pressure with fingertips to the indicated point. Gently press until a deep ache is felt and hold for 30 seconds to a minute. These spots can be pressed as often as needed.

Breech position

Madeline had success with acupuncture: "After a very scary and difficult labor that lasted 40 hours with my son who was 'sunny side up,' I swore I would never do that again. But as everyone warned, I forgot how awful the experience was and we decided to have another baby. When I got pregnant again, I was terrified of giving birth and made my midwives promise that they would check me frequently to make sure the baby was in the correct position before I went into labor. And if the baby wasn't, I wanted to plan a C-section. Sure enough, at seven months, they told me my daughter was breech. The weeks passed, and there was no change. At about eight months, the midwives started encouraging me to think about an ECV (external cephalic version) if the baby didn't turn. I was terrified—I had heard that they were very uncomfortable, not always successful, and (although rare) could hurt the baby. It seemed to me that this was the perfect opportunity to have the 'simple' C-section, but they disagreed. So, we set a date for the ECV, and in the two weeks leading up to it I saw an acupuncturist twice a week for moxibustion. The acupuncturist held a lit mugwort 'cigar' over my pinky toes for a few minutes, until the heat was uncomfortable. I was told it shouldn't hurt, and it didn't. I performed the moxibustion on myself every night at home for two weeks. Finally the day for my ECV came. I was about eight and a half months pregnant, and still terrified. I will never forget the look of amazement on my midwife's face—the baby had turned and was completely in the right position! I was thrilled and almost in disbelief that the baby had turned so late in my pregnancy. To this day, I am absolutely amazed that the acupuncture and moxibustion worked. The experience truly led me to look at alternative and Eastern medicine in a completely different way."

We use a well-known acupuncture and moxibustion protocol to encourage a breech baby to turn, which involves warming a point on the small toe. We must admit that when we first learned about this in graduate school, we were skeptical. It seemed improbable that burning an herb above someone's toe could have any effect on her baby's position. However, over the years we have seen it work over and over again. In fact, it is one of the most tested points in Chinese medicine and has a success rate of anywhere between 69 percent and 85 percent in successive clinical trials.

We usually find that we have better results with this treatment if we see the mom before week 37 of her pregnancy because after that the baby can be too tightly wedged to move. We treat the mom lying on her side and place three or four small acupuncture needles at strategic points. We then use moxa, which is made from an herb—mugwort—that is formed into a stick that looks like a cigar. We hold the smoldering end of the moxa stick above the acupuncture point close to the nail bed of the little toe. We ask the mom to continue to do this for

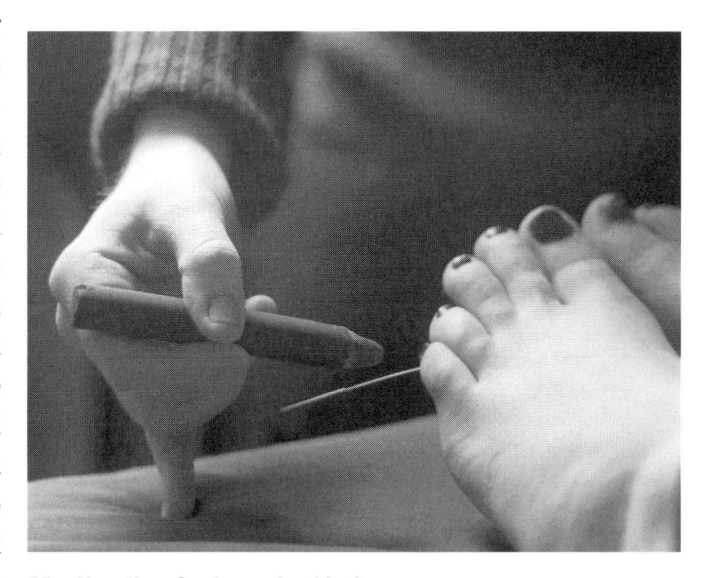

Moxibustion for breeched baby

15 minutes twice a day and we give her moxa sticks to take home so that her partner can do this for her. The feeling is one of relaxing, gentle warmth and should not feel too hot or burn.

The treatment seems to create a bit more space in the uterus, which the baby can use to turn if she feels like it. It may also signal the baby to move and shift position. During the treatment moms tell us that their baby is moving a lot more than usual as they react to the sensation of having more space. If you feel the baby turn, you should stop the treatment and ask your doctor or midwife to check the baby's position.

We like this treatment because it is gentle. If the baby does not turn there may well be a significant reason why not so we prefer that our patients don't do the kind of manipulations that force the baby to turn. The beauty of the moxa treatment is that it only gives the baby more room and does not try and move the baby itself.

Constipation

Because laxatives are not recommended during pregnancy, acupuncture can be a very useful, drug-free way of managing constipation alongside dietary changes. The main point for pregnancy-related constipation (SJ6) is on the arm. It is located about three finger widths up from the wrist in a small depression between the two bones in your arm.

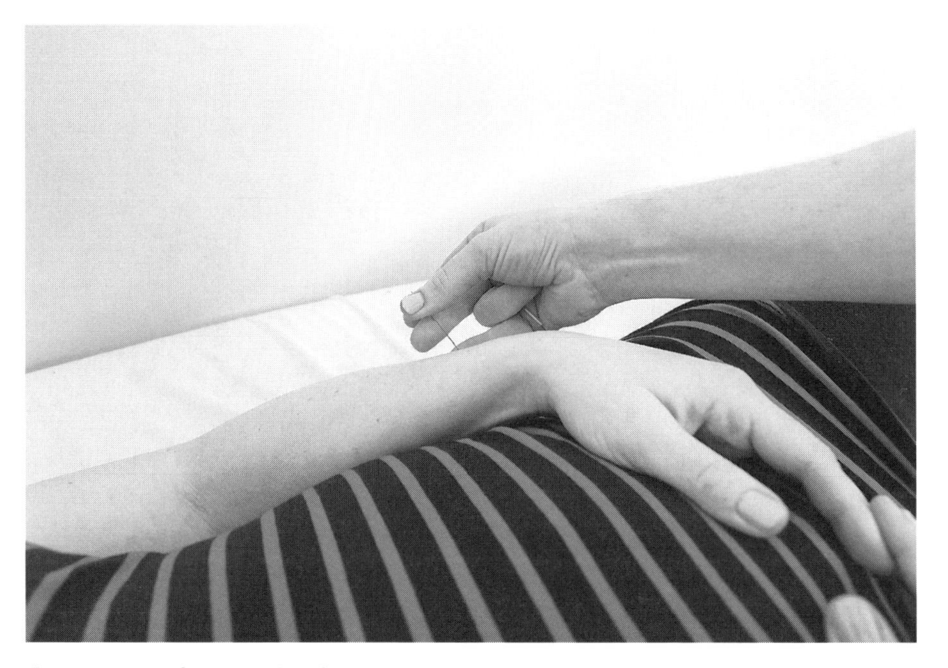

Acupuncture for constipation

Fatigue and anemia

In cases of anemia we do give Chinese herbs as well as suggest diet changes. For fatigue and heaviness of the limbs, we've found acupuncture particularly helpful.

Labor induction

If a patient is past her due date and facing a chemical induction we sometimes do acupuncture to try to help get things started. Some points just above the inner ankle help promote dilation and some points help promote mild contractions. SP6 is located a hands width up from the prominent bone at the inside of the ankle. There is often a slight indentation in the skin, about the size of a pencil eraser, that can be felt at this point.

Morning sickness and nausea

There are different patterns of morning sickness in Chinese medicine and each requires a slightly different approach, but all the acupuncture point prescriptions have one point in common that relieves nausea: PC6.

At YinOva, we needle this point during a treatment and then place magnets on it secured by small sticking plasters. The patient goes home with the magnets attached to keep the treatment going as long as possible. The point is well researched and its efficacy established.

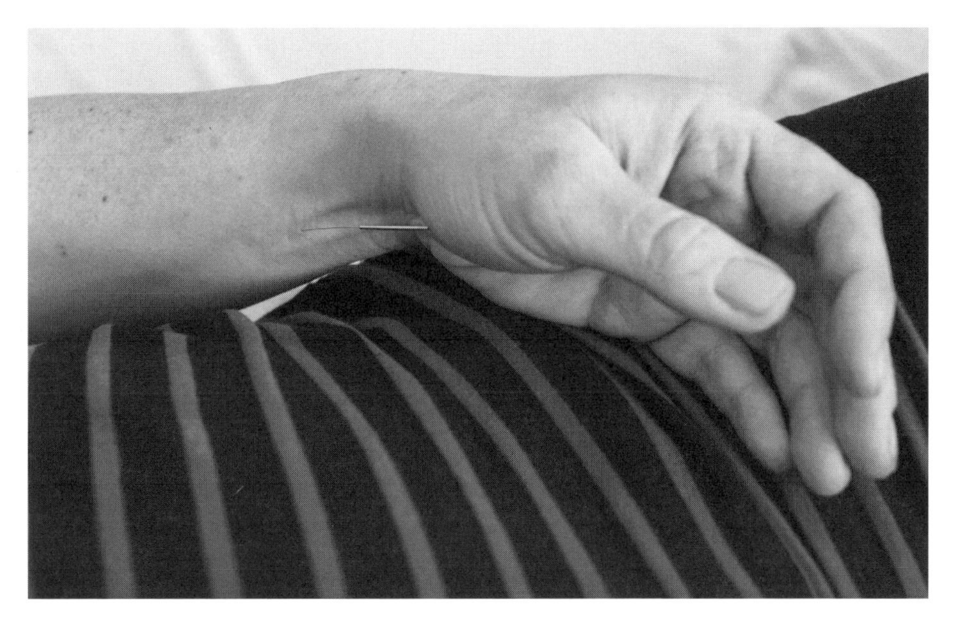

Acupuncture for morning sickness and nausea

You can treat this pressure point on your own. It is located two fingers from your wrist crease, in the center of the wrist, between the two tendons. Gently press until a deep ache is felt and hold for 30 seconds to a minute. This can be done as often as needed to alleviate waves of nausea.

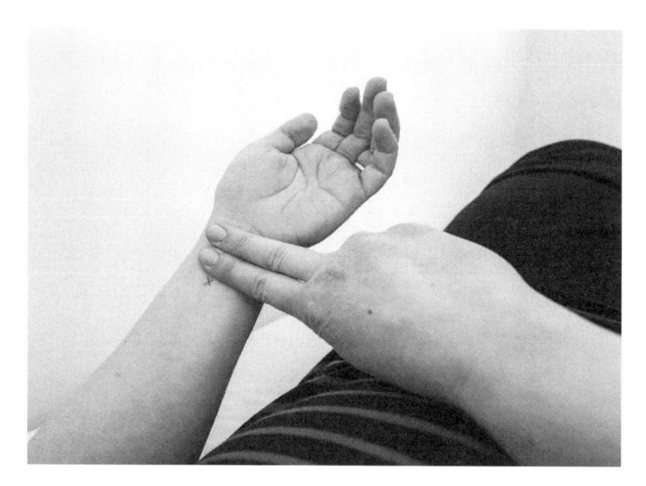

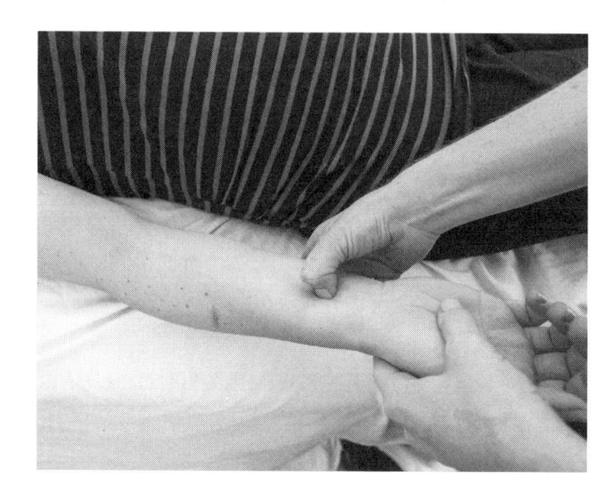

Pressure point for morning sickness and nausea

Musculoskeletal pain

The most common pains we treat with acupuncture are back pain, pelvic pain, rib pain, carpal tunnel syndrome, and leg cramps. All are effectively treated by acupuncture, which is a great choice because it is drug-free. We choose points with different functions to break up muscle spasms, reduce inflammation, interrupt nerve signals, and change the perception of pain in the brain.

Varicose veins, hemorrhoids, and vulvar varicosities

Acupuncture can improve blood flow and reduce the risk of inflammation and clots. Varicosities including hemorrhoids and vulvar varicosities are attributed to central qi dropping in Chinese medicine. We have found treatment to be very effective, with women usually noticing improvement the day after treatment. However, acupuncture isn't necessarily a cure for these conditions. Rather, it provides pain relief and prevents symptoms from worsening as the pregnancy progresses.

Chinese Herbal Medicine

Chinese herbal medicine is used throughout Asia to treat women during pregnancy and postpartum. Usually the herbs are prescribed as custom tailored formulas containing 6 to 15 herbs. At YinOva we try to give pregnant women as few herbs as possible during pregnancy, preferring to use acupuncture as a first-line treatment. However, we do administer herbs for cases of severe morning sickness, edema, headaches, and fatigue. Because each herbal formula is individually tailored it's important to see a board certified herbalist to have a formula specifically designed for you.

We understand you may be struggling during your pregnancy. And you may curse us out when you turn the page and see that we're now telling you to exercise. The next chapter discusses all the myths and truths about exercising for two.

CHAPTER 2

It's Not Time to Put Your Gym Membership on Hold

Shake it up baby, now

We know some of you may be feeling nauseous and lethargic. Exercise is the furthest thing from your mind. But it is important for both you and your baby. So when you muster up the energy, this chapter will address all your questions about exercising during your pregnancy.

If you want to feel better both mentally and physically, then throw on your sneakers and start exercising. You may not be sure what to do. Your mom, boss, and friends are all telling you different things. Plus, what you read on the Internet conflicts with everyone's expert opinion. So who is right? Your doctor or midwife is the ultimate boss, so make sure to clear any exercise plans by him or her first. Sort out the facts from the wives' tales. Here is a list of the myths and rumors you may be getting bombarded with:

1. "Don't Exercise, You Will Hurt the Baby!"

Says who? In a study of almost 1,500 U.S. women, the rate of exercise-related injuries during pregnancy was 4.1 per 1,000 exercise hours. Of these injuries, the majority were bruises or scrapes (55%). That gives you some pretty good odds! You are more likely to hurt yourself by tripping on an uneven sidewalk on your way to the gym. The American Congress of Obstetricians and Gynecologists (ACOG) formally recommend, "In the absence of either medical or obstetric complications, ≥30 minutes of moderate exercise a day on most, if not all, days of the week is recommended for pregnant women." And the benefits? The benefits of physical exercise are infinite. It is hard to find a single individual who wouldn't see health benefits from working up a good sweat. Exercise during pregnancy can benefit your health in the following ways:

- Helps reduce backaches, constipation, bloating, and swelling.
- Helps prevent or treat gestational diabetes.
- Increases your energy and improves your mood.
- Improves your posture.
- Promotes muscle tone, strength, and endurance.
- Helps you sleep better.

Not only can regular exercise help keep you fit during pregnancy and improve your ability to cope with labor, it can also make getting back into shape postbaby much easier.

A new paper by Lehman College Professor Brad Schoenfeld details how even strength training can benefit pregnant women. Professor Schoenfeld is a specialist in exercise science and a faculty member in Lehman's Health Sciences Department.

According to the conclusions he reached after an extensive review of the literature, strength training can reduce the occurrence of gestational diabetes and the severity of both postpartum depression and maternal hypertension, while also easing postpartum weight loss. Other benefits include a 54 percent reduction in the risk of developing preeclampsia during pregnancy (a disorder that can lead to hypertension, edema, and seizures).

Many different types of exercise are safe during pregnancy:

- Walking is a good exercise for anyone.
- Swimming is great for your body because it works so many muscles.
- Cycling provides a good aerobic workout.
- Aerobics is a good way to keep your heart and lungs strong.
- If you were a runner before you became pregnant, you often can keep running during pregnancy, although you may have to modify your routine.

And exercise won't hurt the baby. Quite the contrary! It may actually help the baby. In a large Scandinavian study with almost 6,000 women, sedentary pregnant women were compared with those who participated in more than one type of leisure sports activity. Active women had a significantly reduced risk of preterm birth. Women who engaged in light physical activity (walking) had a 24 percent reduced risk of preterm delivery and women who engaged in moderate to heavy activity (sports such as tennis, swimming, or weekly running, to competitive sports several times a week) had a 66 percent reduced risk.

More Reasons Why Exercising during Pregnancy Is Good for You

Dr. James F. Clapp is an international authority on the effects of exercise during pregnancy. In the early 1980s, he began a series of comprehensive studies that have examined the effects of maternal exercise on the course and outcome of pregnancy. He tracked the effects of frequent (five or more times per week), prolonged (30–90 minutes) bouts of high-intensity (65%–90% of maximum capacity), weight-bearing exercise on competitive runners and aerobic dance instructors. As noted in his book, *Exercising through Your Pregnancy*, babies of women who continued to exercise throughout their pregnancy:

- Tolerated the stress of the contractions much better.
- Had a significantly decreased incidence of cord entanglement.
- Had no difficulty with early weight loss and regained their birth weight rapidly.

Out of more than 250 babies, only four carried by exercising women had obstetrical complications at the start of labor (1%–2%). This was less than that in either the physically active controls (5%) or the women who stopped exercising during their pregnancy (10%).

In almost one hundred offspring at **one year of age**, babies of exercising women did better on standardized intelligence tests. To date, they have done significantly better on the standardized Bayley Scales of Infant Development test than the offspring of the physically active controls. Their mental performance was slightly but significantly better, and their physical performance was better as well.

At **five years of age**, 20 babies born to women who exercised vigorously throughout pregnancy were compared to 20 babies born to women who were physically active controls. The offspring of the women who exercised weighed a little less than the offspring of the physically active. The offspring of the women who exercised scored much higher on tests of general intelligence and oral language skills than the offspring of the physically active controls.

There was a marked decrease in the need for all types of medical intervention for the exercising women. This included:

- A 35 percent decrease in the need for pain relief.
- A 75 percent decrease in the incidence of maternal exhaustion.
- A 50 percent decrease in the need to artificially rupture the membranes.
- A 50 percent decrease in the need to either induce or stimulate labor with Pitocin.
- A 50 percent decrease in the need to intervene because of abnormalities in the fetal heart rate.
- A 55 percent decrease in the need for episiotomy (a cut between vagina and rectum to give the baby more room to deliver).
- A 75 percent decrease in the need for operative intervention (either forceps delivery or cesarean section).

Also:

- Overall weight gain in women that exercised throughout their pregnancy was reduced by 7 pounds.
- More than 65 percent of the exercising women delivered in less than four hours versus 31 percent in the controls.
- The incidence of documented low-back, leg, or pelvic discomfort was less than 10 percent in the exercisers and greater than 40 percent in the controls.

Not only does exercise not hurt the baby, Dr. Allyson Augusta Shrikhande believes that exercise during pregnancy can actually *boost* the baby's brain and cardiovascular development. Dr. Shrikhande of New York Bone and Joint Specialists is a physiatrist who specializes in Women's Health. She states that studies are confirming the positive effects physical activity during pregnancy can have on the baby.

And, given how the physiologies of mother and child intertwine, this has long been suspected.

Dr. Shrikhande states that more and more studies have shown that a baby's heart rate typically rises in unison with his or her exercising mother's, as if the child were also working out! As a result, babies born to active mothers tend to have more robust cardiovascular systems from an early age than babies born to mothers who are more sedentary.

Exercise Is Good for Your Baby Too

Dr. Allyson Augusta Shrikhande reports that the first studies on the effects of exercise on humans and their babies began in 2012 at the University of Montreal in Canada. Researchers recruited a group of local women who were in their first trimester of pregnancy. The women were all healthy, young adults. None were athletes. Few had exercised regularly in the past, and none had exercised more than a day or two per week in the past year. These women were randomized either to begin an exercise program, commencing in their second trimester, or to remain sedentary. The women in the exercise group were asked to work out for at least 20 minutes, three times a week, at a moderate intensity. Most of the women walked or jogged. Every month, for the remainder of each woman's pregnancy, she would visit the university's exercise lab, so researchers could monitor her fitness. All of the volunteers, including those in the nonexercise group, also maintained daily activity logs.

After about six months, the women gave birth to healthy boys or girls. The scientists requested that the mothers almost immediately bring in their children for testing. Within 12 days of birth, each of the newborns accompanied his or her mother to the lab. There, each baby was fitted with a little cap containing electrodes that monitor electrical activity in the brain, settled in his or her mother's lap, and soothed to sleep. Researchers then started a sound loop featuring a variety of low, soft sounds that recurred frequently, interspersed occasionally with more jarring, unfamiliar noises, while the baby's brain activity was recorded. Babies' brains respond to these kinds of sounds with a spike. This spike is most pronounced in immature brains, and diminishes as a newborn's brain develops and begins processing information more efficiently. The spike usually disappears altogether by the time a baby is four months old.

Among the children born to mothers who had remained sedentary during pregnancy, the relevant brainwave "spikes" were large in response to the novel sounds. The brain wave "spikes" were small and blunted in the babies whose mothers had exercised. Therefore, the brains of the babies born to the mothers who had exercised during pregnancy were more mature.

How gestational exercise can remodel an unborn child's brain is not clear. Unlike the circulatory systems, a mother's brain is not directly connected to that of her child. In the medical community, we suspect that when mothers exercise in pregnancy, they generate a variety of chemicals that move into her bloodstream and eventually mingle with the blood of her baby. These chemicals affect the brain development of the child.

If a woman can be physically active during her pregnancy, she may give her unborn child an advantage, in terms of brain development.

You do, however, have a legitimate excuse to bench yourself from some activities. Collision sports, such as hockey and basketball, should be avoided, as should sports with a high incidence of falling, such as skiing and horseback riding. Since a protective cup for your belly hasn't yet been invented, you need to avoid the risk of trauma to your baby through a direct blow or fall. Tuck those riding boots and skates away for a few more months.

If you have abdominal pain while exercising that is lasting longer than a few seconds, you should contact your doctor or midwife immediately. It may be from preterm labor, preeclampsia, placental abruption, or a medical problem unrelated to pregnancy.

When else should you throw in the towel? The American College of Sports Medicine (ACSM) lists several reasons to discontinue exercise and seek medical advice during pregnancy:

1. Any signs of bloody discharge from the vagina.
2. Any "gush" of fluid from the vagina (premature rupture of membranes).
3. Sudden swelling of the ankles, face, or hands.
4. Persistent, severe headaches and/or visual disturbance; unexplained spell of faintness or dizziness.
5. Swelling, pain, and redness in the calf of one leg (phlebitis).
6. Elevation of pulse rate or blood pressure that persists after exercise.

7. Excessive fatigue, palpitations, chest pain.
8. Persistent contractions (more than 6–8 per hour) that may suggest onset of premature labor.
9. Unexplained abdominal pain.
10. Insufficient weight gain (less than 1.0 kilograms or 2.2 pounds per month) during the last two trimesters.

These can be the signs of dangerous medical conditions during pregnancy. You should see your doctor or midwife immediately for an evaluation should these symptoms occur.

Medical Guidelines for Pregnant Athletes

The American Congress of Obstetrics and Gynecology states that female athletes who participated in athletics and exercise programs prior to their pregnancy should continue to do so provided their pregnancy remains uncomplicated. So if you're looking for a reason not to exercise, you can't use this one!

Paula Radcliffe, the world record holder in the women's marathon, ran throughout two pregnancies. Ms. Radcliffe ran twice a day during the first five months of her pregnancy in 2006, then cut back as she approached her due date. She was the first female finisher in the 2007 New York City marathon, just ten months after her daughter was born.

We know professional athletes have teams of coaches, doctors, trainers, nutritionists, and support staff to help them, but don't let pregnancy prevent you from staying active. You don't need to be superwoman, either. Make sure to talk to your doctor about your exercise regimen; pregnancy is no reason to automatically throw in the towel, but you do want to avoid certain dangerous sport activities. Scuba diving and water skiing, for example, are not safe for you or the baby.

2. "If You Have Pain While Exercising during the Beginning of Your Pregnancy, Stop Everything Because It's Only Going to Get Worse."

Not necessarily! Your body changes throughout your pregnancy. Each week something new happens. For example, your fluctuating pregnancy hormones may be your worst enemy one week and your best friend the next. Its role in pregnancy is to prepare your body for the growing baby's occupancy and delivery. Your pregnancy hormones allow your ligaments and joints to loosen and expand to make room for your growing uterus and pelvis. These adaptations facilitate your baby's descent down the birth canal. These hormones also allow your blood vessels to widen to accommodate the increased blood flow you and your baby need during pregnancy. These levels peak during the first 14 weeks of pregnancy and again at the time of delivery.

Some women love the effects of their increasing pregnancy hormones and others loathe it. If you've always struggled with poor flexibility and stiffness, you may embrace this newly found mobility. It is time to move up to the front of your prenatal yoga class and show off your poses! In contrast, some of you may feel more out of alignment and unstable from the changes in your joint laxity. You may twist your ankle or throw out your back when your joints are looser. It will be helpful for you to partake in exercises that work both sides of your body equally, such as walking, running, cycling, or swimming. And remember, these elevated hormone levels will decrease after your first trimester, so don't write off exercises that may feel too uncomfortable, as they may become easier.

You may also have pain from your uterine ligaments in your second trimester, but this too will change. There are several ligaments supporting your growing uterus. These ligaments stretch as your uterus expands and tightens up with sudden movements. In the nonpregnant woman, the uterus is an almost-solid structure weighing about 70 grams (or 1.5 pounds) and with a cavity of 10 milliliters (or 2 teaspoons) or less. During pregnancy, the uterus is transformed into a relatively thin-walled muscular organ of sufficient capacity to accommodate the fetus, placenta, and amnionic fluid. The total volume of the contents at term averages about 5 liters but may be 20 liters (about five gallons) or more. By the end of pregnancy, the uterus has achieved a capacity that is 500 to 1,000 times greater than in the nonpregnant state. That equals approximately 1,100 grams (or 2.4 pounds)!

Your round ligament is often the culprit for the abdominal pain during your second trimester. Refer to the section in Chapter 1 on round ligament pain for ways to reduce round ligament discomfort.

The shape of your uterus is constantly changing during pregnancy, from elongated to oval to round and then back to oval, which will affect the surrounding organs and soft tissues. As the uterus grows and expands, the ligaments attached to the uterus get stretched. Nerve fibers that run next to the ligaments stretch along with them and can cause pain.

The uterus also moves around as it increases in size. It migrates up into the abdomen by the fourth month. This takes some pressure off of your ligaments, but this position makes breathing more challenging. So your ligaments feel better, but you can't breathe. Sorry! To breathe easier you'll have to wait for your uterus to drop down again, toward the end of your third trimester at week 36.

During your second trimester, you will also experience some muscle soreness from your recent weight gain, change in posture, and new demands on your body. Should this happen, please let your doctor or midwife know. It may be a musculoskeletal issue that can easily be addressed by a physical therapist or other health care provider.

3. "Don't Let Your Heart Rate Get Higher than 140 Beats Per Minute When Exercising. And Don't Exercise for More than 15 Minutes."

This "rule" was written in 1985, but then amended in 1994 by the American Congress of Obstetricians and Gynecologists. However, many health care providers and institutions still follow this antiquated guideline. James F. Clapp III, MD, has been the world's foremost researcher in the area of exercise and pregnancy since the early 1980s. It was based on his findings that this addendum was added in 1994 eliminating the 140 beats per minute heart rate rule and guiding women to use the "talk-test" as a way to measure intensity. The "talk-test" is when the expecting mother works out at an intensity where she can speak three- to five-word sentences. Anything less, they are working out too hard; anything more, they can pick up the pace within their comfort level. Also, note that studies that were first done to determine appropriate heart rates for pregnant females were performed on pregnant female *animals*. It was only recently that studies started taking into account pregnant *human* females. This may be a good reason why guidelines keep changing.

So how do you know how hard to work out? What are the current guidelines? You need to measure how you feel, not what your heart rate monitor reads. You should be able to hold a conversation and not feel overheated or out of breath. If you can't speak normally while you're working out, you're probably pushing yourself too hard. This could lead to vaginal bleeding, uterine contractions, or other problems, according to Dr. Roger W. Harms of the Mayo Clinic. While there have been no studies looking specifically at the effects of intense training on pregnancy, guidelines set by the federal Department of Health and Human Services say that women can sustain the level of physical activity they engaged in prior to pregnancy. Make sure to keep your body cool by staying hydrated and wearing loose or moisture-wicking clothing.

4. "It's Not Safe to Ride a Bike after Your First Trimester."

This depends on your comfort level while cycling, the size of your belly, and your ability to pedal underneath your growing belly. Balance is affected during pregnancy by the change in your posture and center of gravity. Your back starts to curve more with your protruding belly. The over-stretched core muscles lose their strength and balance is more difficult to obtain. This may cause you to be unsafe while riding a mountain or road bike outdoors. There are many variables outside your control, such as dogs, children and cars. You may not have the strength and coordination to avoid these obstacles. *The BMJ* reports there is no increased incidence of falls in pregnant women, but we don't want you to take the chance. As your pregnancy progresses, we recommend cycling indoors for optimal safety. And if you fall off a stationary bike, we will give you a get-out-of-gym-card for free. Just stay safe!

5. "Too Much Exercise Will Take Nutrients Away from Your Baby."

Some believe that exercise reduces the rate of oxygen and nutrient delivery to the developing fetus as the body shunts blood away from internal organs to supply the exercising muscles. This won't happen. The normal physiologic adaptation to pregnancy is increased cardiac output and blood volume. This additional blood flow constitutes a significant portion of your pregnancy weight gain. Additionally, the placenta (the organ that connects the baby to the mom's blood supply) is designed to ensure constant nutrient delivery during a healthy pregnancy. There is no retrospective evidence to suggest that exercise leads to fetal distress, premature delivery, or low birth weight.

6. "If You Never Exercised before Pregnancy, Don't Start Now."

Don't listen to these people. The American Congress of Obstetrics and Gynecology (ACOG) encourages pregnant women to be evaluated before starting a new exercise program and participating in low-impact activities. Stretching, walking, pelvic floor exercises, and breathing exercises are also safe. Besides the psychological health benefits of feeling better, releasing stress, sleeping better, and clearing your head, women show physical improvements in their cardiovascular endurance, blood pressure levels, body fat index, muscular strength and endurance, and maximum heart rate.

A supervised and structured exercise regimen provides little if any risk to the mom or baby. That being said, pregnancy isn't a time to be ultra-competitive. It's a time to take care of yourself and the little one in your belly.

7. "Avoid All Forms of Prenatal Yoga."

There are many benefits to practicing yoga. Some studies show lowered rates in depression and anxiety during pregnancy. Yoga helps to develop strength and improve balance, as well as teaches you to breathe properly.

Some cautions, however. Some yoga poses recommend spending time on your hands and knees ("on all fours") or in plank (push-up) position. This may feel great for your back but can be too strenuous on your abdominal connective tissue and muscles. In this position, the weight of your organs and expanding uterus can strain the soft tissue between your abdominal muscles. Exercising in this position can cause an abdominal separation (diastasis recti) or worsen one that you already have (and may not know of). We encourage you to avoid these positions. Spend minimal time in these positions and more time sitting or standing in yoga class. (Please see the section on diastasis recti in Chapter 1).

Certain yoga positions may also call for you to lean back or extend your spine (curve it backwards). Stretches that are on your hands and knees (such as "cat/camel" stretch), on your stomach (such as "cobra"), or in a sitting position to open up your chest require you to curve your spine backwards. During pregnancy, your spine is *already* under the influence of increased weight from the front of your body, causing it to curve backwards. The weight of your growing baby pulls forward on the spine and puts a lot of stress on the ligaments and discs. You may have noticed this change in your posture already. You want to minimize any more forward stress and avoid movements that require you to bend backwards. Try to keep your spine as straight or neutral as you can when you exercise.

There are many yoga poses that challenge your balance (such as tree pose). These are great to practice for stability. However, always keep in mind that your center of gravity or point of balance in your body is constantly shifting as your pregnancy progresses. As with all exercises during pregnancy, start slow and see how your body adjusts to new movements. Make sure there is something sturdy nearby to grab in case you lose your balance. Attractive class participants are not excluded!

Have your friends told you to not do hot yoga? Your friends are right. There have not been any studies published on the effects of increased body temperature (from a grueling Bikram or hot yoga class) on the developing baby; however, we know it is important to regulate your body temperature during pregnancy to avoid preterm labor, and this is hard to accomplish in a room that is 105 degrees Fahrenheit and about 40 percent humidity.

You want to stay cool while exercising and can accomplish this by avoiding outdoor exercise for extended periods in hot/humid weather; wearing loose layered clothes that can be removed as your body warms up; drinking plenty of fluids before, during, and after you exercise; and controlling your intensity by monitoring how you feel. You should be exercising at an intensity that allows you to hold a conversation with a friend (or yourself!)

8. "You Shouldn't Stretch during Pregnancy. Your Joints Are Too Loose."

Yes, your joints are a little looser during pregnancy, thanks to your elevated hormones. However, that doesn't mean you shouldn't stretch. The connective tissue in your body is under the influence of hormones called relaxin, progesterone, and estrogen. And guess what relaxin does? It relaxes! Its job is to relax the connective tissue in and around the pelvis to allow the baby to grow and be delivered. The problem with relaxin (along with your increasing levels of progesterone and estrogen) is that it doesn't just go to work in the pelvis. These hormones that get released affect all connective tissue in the body. So they do make your joints looser, which can ultimately lead to instability issues. These hormones don't cause pain, but they initiate the sequence that does. This can lead to instability of a joint, which can lead to dysfunctions, which can then lead to painful symptoms.

So what does this mean? It means a few things: It could mean that if you like to jog, you may have to be careful with regard to which surfaces you run on. If you are running on an uneven surface, your ankles may not be stable enough to support your body if your foot accidentally lands on a crack in the sidewalk. This could lead to a sprain or strain injury.

What does this mean for stretching? You don't want to be too aggressive with your stretching, but you can definitely stretch your muscles and joints. Hold your stretches for 30 seconds and make sure you feel a comfortable "pull" in the muscle or joint. Don't overdo it, though. For safe stretches for your muscles and joints, see Chapter 1.

9. "Running Is Too Jarring for the Baby"

You may worry that the baby will get hurt if you do too much high-impact exercise. You may think that the baby will not tolerate the movement or that the movement may set off preterm labor. Don't worry, the baby won't be injured and he or she won't fall out. The baby is more protected and cushioned than you may think. If anything, *you* have to make sure that *you* are protected when you exercise. Remember those pregnancy hormones that are making your joints looser? You have to make sure that you keep an eye on the surfaces that you are running on so you don't step on an uneven surface and risk spraining your ankle. Also, remember that as your belly grows, you won't be able to see your feet! Make sure your laces are tied properly and that your shoes are a comfortable fit for your swollen feet.

Just make sure you are cleared by your doctor or midwife before starting an exercise program, especially if you want to maintain a high level of activity.

Exercise during Fertility Treatments

Strenuous exercise while undergoing fertility treatments should be avoided, as an ovarian torsion, the rotation or twisting of an enlarged ovary, cutting off its blood and venous supply, causing severe abdominal pain and necrosis (premature death of body tissue), is an unwanted possibility.

When undergoing fertility treatments, a woman will take medications to hyper-stimulate her ovaries and increase follicle production. These follicles contain eggs, and one (or more) will open to release an egg during ovulation each month. The follicles that fail to open remain in the ovaries and become follicular cysts. While housing these cysts, the ovaries aren't able to resume their original size and remain enlarged.

Strenuous activity can cause torsion of the swollen ovaries. This can occur when the ovary gets twisted, often with the fallopian tube. Blood flow to the ovary gets occluded in the twisted structures. Without adequate blood flow, the ovary won't survive and often needs to be surgically removed. An ultrasound will determine if you have remaining cysts after your treatment, and your reproductive endocrinologist will guide you accordingly. The cysts usually go away after a menstrual cycle or pregnancy.

We know fertility treatments are stressful and running is a great stress-release, but this is a serious condition you want to avoid. So be smart and follow your doctor's instructions, please!

10. "Don't Lift That, It's Too Heavy."

You can respond to this statement in two ways:

1. You can say, "Yes! you're right!" and milk the situation for all it's worth.

2. You can gauge the weight of the object (or child) you are lifting, use proper body mechanics, breathe properly, and use a maternity belt if necessary.

Research suggests not lifting more than 15 to 20 pounds during pregnancy. Whoever established this guideline clearly doesn't have a rambunctious toddler to chase! And you can't always execute the perfect body mechanics to lift your child who may be squirming around as you lift him or her. So do your best when the occasion arises. Don't be afraid to grab some help if you feel that what/who you are lifting is too heavy. Remember, this is no time to be superwoman if you don't have to be.

According to the Cleveland Clinic, here are some tips to keep in mind when lifting something:

- If you must lift objects, do not try to lift objects that are awkward or are heavier than 20 pounds. (Again, we understand that your older child is probably more than 20 pounds. Do your best to minimize your lifting loads.)
- Before you lift an object, make sure you have firm footing.
- To pick up an object that is lower than the level of your waist, keep your back straight and bend at your knees and hips. Do not bend forward at the waist with your knees straight.
- Stand with a wide stance close to the object you are trying to pick up, and keep your feet firmly on the ground. Tighten your stomach muscles along with your pelvic floor muscles and lift the object using your leg muscles. Straighten your knees in a steady motion. Don't jerk the object up to your body.
- Stand completely upright without twisting. Always move your feet forward when lifting an object.
- If you are lifting an object from a table, slide it to the edge of the table so you can hold it close to your body. Bend your knees so you are close to the object. Use your legs to lift the object and come to a standing position.
- Avoid lifting heavy objects above waist level.
- Hold packages close to your body with your arms bent. Keep your stomach muscles tight. Take small steps and go slowly.
- To lower the object, place your feet as you did to lift. Tighten your stomach muscles, and bend your hips and knees.

If you feel that you need some extra stabilization, you can wear a maternity belt or support. These belts, when applied properly, can offer extra stability and assist you with your lifting. They also serve as a mental reminder to protect your back while lifting and use correct body mechanics.

While we remind you not to lift with your back, it doesn't mean you shouldn't lift weights or do some form of strength training during your pregnancy. Remember, you will soon have a 10 pound weight glued to your hip. This new addition will test your quads and biceps and you'll be doing a lot of squats. So be prepared. If you don't have a gym membership, you can use your body weight and do some squats and wall push-ups. (See page 6 for how to do squats against a wall and page 16 for how to do wall push-ups). Grab some light hand weights, resistance bands, or objects found around your home, such as filled water bottles, for some upper body strengthening. You can even exercise from the confines of your bed. You want to be ready to carry that infant around … and the car seat, and the stroller, and the diaper bag, and the laundry basket with a baby in it, and....

11. "You Should Be Able to Maintain a Conversation While Exercising."

Absolutely. If you are out of breath and can't talk, you and your baby may not be getting enough oxygen. Being able to maintain a conversation while exercising is an important gauge for determining whether or not you are working out too hard. This actually is called the "talk test." The American Congress of Sports Medicine reports that this is a good way to monitor exercise intensity during pregnancy. If you are exercising, even at a higher level of activity, you shouldn't be gasping for air or overheating. You should be able to talk to a friend at a comfortable level and exchange proper gossip. If you are unable to speak full sentences during your exercise routine, slow down, take long slow deep breaths, and decrease the intensity of your workout. And if you're able to sing the *Rocky IV* soundtrack, then step it up a notch. Just think how proud you will be that you and your friend exercised together instead of going out for cupcakes.

How Hard Should You Be Working Out?

In late pregnancy (30 weeks plus), because of changes in your blood volume, you're going to struggle to get your heart rate up to what you think it should be, unless you're working extremely hard. So how can you monitor yourself if heart rate is not an ideal indicator?

Throughout pregnancy, a more reliable measure to use is the Borg CR10 Scale. Using the Borg scale, you rate your perception of exertion on a scale of 0 to 10, with 1 to 2 meaning able to converse with no effort, 5 meaning some effort required for talking, and 9 to 10 meaning talking is impossible. You should be rating your perceived exertion at around Level 5 when you are working out. Use this scale along with the Talk Test to monitor your workout.

12. "Drinking Eight Glasses of Water Is Enough, Even When You Exercise."

We know the scenario. You're constantly running to the bathroom and your limbs resemble sausage links from all the water you're retaining. The last thing you want to do is drink more water. However, keeping properly hydrated is essential during pregnancy. Adequate hydration maintains a healthy internal body temperature and fluid volume necessary during pregnancy. If the nonpregnant person is drinking eight glasses of water a day, you should be drinking closer to 10 to 12 glasses of water each day.

You should not wait until you feel thirsty to drink water. Thirst is a sign of dehydration. You should consistently be drinking water throughout the day. When you exercise, you have to drink even more water. It is recommended that pregnant women drink:

- 16 ounces of fluid two hours before exercising.
- 8 to 16 ounces of fluid 10 to 15 minutes prior to exercise.
- 3 to 10 ounces every 10 to 20 minutes during exercise.
- 1 pint of water for every pound lost during your exercise routine.

You also have to consider increasing your water intake if you are exercising outside on a warm day. Just make sure there is a restroom nearby so you don't have to worry about accidents!

Now that you are ready to exercise, we need to address your pelvic floor. Peeing when you run or jump isn't much fun, so let's talk about how to take care of the muscles down there next.

C H A P T E R 3

Help for the Pelvic Floor

I laughed so hard I just peed in my pants

Holly told us her pelvic floor weakness began during her last pregnancy two years ago and never improved. She has avoided high impact exercise classes and running, which she enjoyed pre-pregnancy. She stays far away from bouncy houses and trampolines, as she knows her body can't tolerate the jumping. She is now 14 weeks pregnant and wears pads every day to avoid embarrassing leaks. She does Kegels every day while commuting to work, but doesn't see a difference. She is worried she will eventually need a diaper and she is only 39 years old.

Your pelvic floor muscles act as a sling that supports your pelvis in several ways. They support your pelvic organs (bladder, uterus, rectum), give stability to your pelvis, and contribute to sexual and bladder/bowel function. Your doctor, midwife, or friends may have already told you to "do your Kegels!" to strengthen your pelvic floor. We know you want to ignore this advice, but you shouldn't. Or you will pee in your pants.

But do you really know where your Kegel muscles are? Do you know *what* your Kegel muscles are? Most women think they do. When asked to do a Kegel contraction, they squeeze every muscle in their body, hold their breath, and turn red. But they skip their pelvic floors. Try it. Go ahead and squeeze your pelvic floor muscles for five seconds. Are you breathing? Are you squeezing your butt muscles? Did you squeeze your knees together? Are you sucking in your stomach? Are you flattening your back? Then you are not doing proper Kegel exercises. They're tricky, aren't they?

Read on for everything you need to know to do a proper Kegel. Trust us, it's worth the effort to keep these muscles strong. Strong pelvic floor muscles will be your friend throughout the pregnancy. Remember that by the end of pregnancy, the uterus has achieved a capacity that is 500 to 1000 times greater than in the nonpregnant state. Your pelvic floor has to support this enormous growth! Healthy pelvic floor muscles will also help you to not leak as much during and after your pregnancy. Recovering faster after you have the baby will also be easier if you are working these muscles during pregnancy.

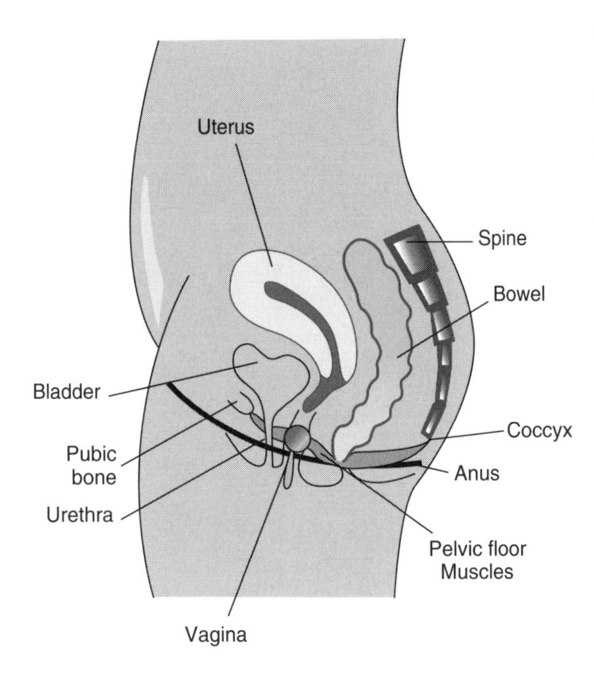

What's a Kegel?

Dr. Arnold Henry Kegel (a man!) first identified exercises to target the pelvic floor muscles in the 1940s. These exercises as well as the pelvic floor muscles were named after him. So the "Kegel muscles" are actually your levator ani muscles. (Clearly not as catchy as "Kegel muscles.") These particular pelvic floor muscles are just one component lining the base of your pelvis.

The Love Boat

Here's a way to think a little differently about your pelvic floor muscles. Imagine that your pelvic organs (bladder, uterus, rectum) are represented by a floating boat in a dock. The water underneath the boat represents the pelvic floor muscles supporting the boat from underneath. The ropes tying the boat to the dock represent the connective tissue and ligaments that are anchoring the pelvic organs to the pelvic wall, which is located just below your abdominal wall.

When the water levels are not adequate under the boat, there is increased tension on the ropes tying the boat to the dock. There could even be a lot of pressure from one part of the boat to another, especially if the water levels are uneven or choppy under the boat. So if the pelvic floor muscles are weak, there could be a lot of stress on the connective tissues/ligaments anchoring the pelvic organs. And there could be pressure from one pelvic organ onto another. Now imagine all the increased pressure from your growing uterus on the neighboring pelvic organs. If there is enough water underneath the boat, then the boat is sufficiently supported. The goal is to keep the pelvic floor muscles strong and healthy so all the pelvic organs and their connective tissues are not overly strained and too tight.

Pelvic Floor Muscles and Bowel and Bladder Function

There are many layers of pelvic floor muscles. The levator ani (Kegel) muscles are big sheets of muscles that wrap around the base of your pelvic organs—bladder, vagina, and rectum. So when you squeeze these muscles, you are essentially closing off the organs, which then stop you from leaking. If you cough, laugh, sneeze, jump, or lift something heavy (including your new baby), you increase the pressure in your abdomen. This increased pressure then stresses your organs, which can lead you to leak urine, stool, or gas. This is called "stress incontinence." Your new baby won't be the only one who needs diapers!

Your body should reflexively tighten these pelvic floor muscles to close off the organs so you don't leak. You shouldn't have to think about it. However, sometimes your muscles get weak and they forget what they are supposed to do. Maybe they get pregnancy brain also. The increasing weight and size of your uterus will put additional pressure on both your pelvic floor and bladder. So you have to work extra hard to remind these pelvic floor muscles to support your organs.

Pelvic Floor Muscles and Sexual Function

There are many fabulous reasons to have sex, but did you know that there are therapeutic health benefits from getting it on? The different layers of the pelvic floor muscles wrap around the vagina as well as connect right to the clitoris. They contribute directly to sexual function by contracting around the vagina and lifting the hood of the clitoris during orgasm. Not only does a strong pelvic floor increase sexual pleasure, but when the pelvic floor muscles are well toned, they are able to contract and relax more; this helps to build more arousal, intensify sexual sensations, and increase your ability to control your orgasms.

When you voluntarily contract your pelvic floor muscles, you are keeping these sexual functioning muscles healthy. They need exercise too! In Chapter 4, we will discuss different sexual positions, how to accommodate your pregnant belly during sex, and other sex-related issues. Just know that keeping these muscles strong also ensures an enjoyable sex life.

Pelvic Floor Muscles and Your Pelvic Stability

When people think about hip, butt, or pelvic muscles, they mainly think about muscles that are on the "outside." You know, like those infamous gluteus maximus muscles. However, the muscles on the inside are just as important. They sometimes get ignored simply because they cannot be seen when they contract. Not only do these internal pelvic floor muscles contribute to sexual, bladder, and bowel function, they also contribute to the stability of your pelvis. They attach to your tailbone, as well as the other bones in your pelvis. So if your muscles are weak or tight you may experience uneven forces pulling on your pelvis. This can affect your pregnant posture, the way you walk, and the pain you may feel. Pain may pop up in your tailbone since the muscles attach there. Or you may feel discomfort in your hips, low abdomen, or in the back or front of your pelvis.

Underactive and Overactivepelvic Floor Dysfunction

You may fall into one of two categories. You may have an "overactive pelvic floor dysfunction" or an "underactive pelvic floor dysfunction." They both sound geriatric and scary, but they're not. Your pelvic floor muscles are either too weak or too tight.

With underactive pelvic floor muscles, you may experience leaking of urine, feces, or gas because the muscles are not contracting properly to close off your bladder or rectum.

With overactive pelvic floor muscles, you may experience pain in your pelvis because the muscles are too tight and can't relax. Just what you want: a Type-A pelvic floor. The muscles are always "on guard," which can lead to painful spasms or trigger points. Trigger points are tight spots or "knots" in muscles. They can feel very tender when pressed. They can even refer pain to other regions of the body if they are intense and have been around for a while.

Learning how to efficiently use your pelvic floor muscles will help you. You want good pelvic control so you can recruit these muscles when you need them and relax them when you don't.

Pregnancy and the Pelvic Floor

You might be wondering if your pelvic floor is even still functioning when you are nine months pregnant. It is! It may be a little harder to recruit the muscles as they are under a lot of stress, literally. Your baby (or babies) is/are getting bigger and that places more pressure on the muscles supporting it. Your recent pregnancy pounds cause your center of gravity to shift forward. So if you feel like you are going to fall on your face, it isn't just because you're exhausted from not sleeping well. Plus, your joints are a little looser with your elevated pregnancy hormones. All these factors put more stress on the pelvic floor. And if these muscles aren't strong enough, you are more prone to leaking. If the muscles get too tight from being over-taxed, you are more susceptible to pain and injury.

Now we are ready to learn how to train these muscles to help you stay dry and pain free.

How to Strengthen Your Pelvic Floor

First, we have to *FIND* these muscles.

Let's try to use some simple visual biofeedback to find these muscles. All you will need is a handheld mirror. Get into a comfortable position. You can lie down in your bed and bend your knees. Use pillows to prop up your back so you are not flat. Now don't be shy. If you haven't already been introduced, please meet your vagina. Take your handheld mirror and angle it so that you can see the area between your vagina and anus. This area is called your "perineum."

Before you start, make sure you don't have to go to the bathroom. Strengthening the muscles is easier with an empty bladder.

Now, take a deep breath and as you exhale, try to squeeze your pelvic floor muscles. Imagine you just drank a venti decaf Starbucks coffee. You're stuck in a meeting and you really have to pee. Tighten your muscles as if you're holding your urine.

Looking into the mirror, do you see the area between your vagina and anus move up and inward toward your body? Is there any movement at all? If you are contracting your muscles correctly, then you will see this occur. Try again! Try and relax all of your other muscles and just focus on that area.

I Still Can't Find the Muscles! What Do You Mean I Have to Breathe at the Same Time?

Don't worry! Let's try again.

Go ahead and sit at the edge of your bed. Sit on a small rolled-up hand towel, along the length of your pelvic floor.

Focus on your breathing and make sure to not hold your breath.

Contract your pelvic floor muscles as you exhale. Try to squeeze your muscles up and in. Imagine you are picking up the towel with your perineum. Relax your thighs and your stomach. I know you are concentrating very hard but I don't want you to cheat.

Now relax the muscles and put down the towel.

Grrr. No Luck. I Still Can't Connect with Them

Then you need us! Ask your doctor or midwife for a referral to a women's health physical therapist. We can help you locate the correct muscles. Biofeedback is a helpful tool to see the muscle activity. With biofeedback, small sticker electrodes can be placed on your pelvic floor muscles near your anus. These sensors pick up your muscle activity. The sensors have leads that connect to a computer and you can see what your muscles are doing on the screen. If there isn't a clear difference on the screen when you are contracting and relaxing your muscles, your physical therapist will help you. It may be easier for you to contract the muscles from a different position, while co-contracting other hip or core muscles, or by coordinating your breaths with your contractions. Some women respond better to an internal vaginal sensor. The internal sensor won't pick up external muscle activity if you're compensating with adjacent muscles. So it makes it harder to cheat. You will need to have your doctor or midwife clear you for this first.

It's OK if you can't get a good contraction right away. Just like any other skeletal muscle in your body, strengthening takes time. If you lifted a 10-pound dumbbell in your hand a few times, you wouldn't look like Popeye after the first few repetitions. These muscles are hard to recruit because you can't see them. But don't be discouraged!

OK, I've Found the Muscles. How Do I Get Them Stronger?

If you were working out at the gym, how would you strengthen your thigh muscles? You would find the machine where you sit and lift a bar that's supported by the front of your lower legs. You would do that 10 times. Then rest and do it again another 10 times. Then maybe you would do something functional such as squatting to target your thigh muscles. Correct? We have to think of the pelvic floor muscles the same way. We need to strengthen them through repetition and recruit them when we are doing functional movements. So let's begin.

Once you think you have the right muscles isolated, try these exercises.

Lying down: squeezing for as long as you can

Squeeze 10 times. Hold it for as long as you can sustain a good contraction. This may only be two to three seconds long. Shoot for

10 seconds but make sure you aren't compensating and using all your adjacent muscles. Don't hold your breath.

Rest.

Repeat again 10 times.

Rest.

Lying down: quick squeezes

Sometimes you leak when you are trying to get to the bathroom that's all the way at the end of the hallway. Sometimes you leak when you cough, laugh, sneeze, or lift something. Why is this happening?

There are different fibers in the pelvic floor muscles that recruit during different times. When you sneeze, your quick recruiting fibers kick in. When you are stuck on a long bus ride, your endurance fibers kick in to hold in your urine. So you need to exercise both sets of these fibers. You have to exercise the *whole* muscle.

In addition to squeezing for as long as you can, practice squeezing just for one second and fully relaxing for one second. These contractions are called "quick squeezes." You are exercising the quick recruiting fibers. Repeat this 10 times in a row. If this is easy, try another 10 repetitions.

Now that you can contract your pelvic floor muscles while you are lying down, try sitting up and squeezing.

Sitting

Your muscles will feel different in this different position. Gravity and the baby are pushing down on your muscles now. You can also practice this while sitting on a large exercise ball. Lean forward slightly and let your legs be wider than hip-width apart. You should be able to feel your muscles contract and relax against the surface of the ball. This sensation should let you know if you are doing the exercises right. The large exercise ball will also come in handy later when you are in labor. This will be described in Chapter 6.

You can strengthen your pelvic muscles while getting up from a chair.

Getting up from a chair

Try transitioning from sitting to standing. Don't forget to squeeze your muscles *while* you are changing positions. When you change positions, the pressure in your abdomen also changes and this will affect your bladder. If you squeeze as you stand up from a sitting position, you can prevent leaking and train the muscles to be stronger and more effective.

Standing

Now that you are standing, notice how different it feels to squeeze your muscles in this position. The baby is really putting pressure on your muscles and it may feel very hard to recruit the muscles. But you can do it! Don't forget to breathe, please.

Practice both your endurance contractions and quick squeezes. Try squeezing the muscles for as long as you can and also for one second at a time in this standing position.

Make sure you are standing next to something sturdy that you can hold on to in case you feel off balance when you move on to the next set of exercises.

Try challenging the muscles by kicking your leg out to the side or behind you while you are squeezing your pelvic floor muscles. Try marching or performing little mini squats. Be aware of maintaining your pelvic floor muscle contraction throughout the exercise. Do 10 repetitions of each exercise.

You may feel these little muscles fatiguing. Give yourself a break once this occurs. If your muscles are too fatigued to fire, you will start compensating by recruiting other muscles. This is cheating, so just take a break and resume when your pelvic floor muscles can correctly perform another set.

Don't be hard on yourself if you have a difficult time recruiting your pelvic floor muscles. Every month, the baby is getting bigger and putting more pressure on your bladder and muscles. It's going to be progressively challenging, but don't get discouraged. Keep practicing and your hard work will pay off.

When Should I Do These Exercises?

The beauty of doing your Kegel exercises is that no one knows when you are doing them. You can squeeze away while on the train, while waiting on line at the post office, or while watching TV. You don't need equipment, just a little attention to your pelvis.

You can practice exercising your pelvic muscles all day, every day. But more importantly, what are you doing when you leak? Do you drip a little when you pick up your baby or the laundry basket? What about when you stand up after sitting for a while? Think about what you do during the day and when your pelvic floor feels the weakest. Try squeezing your pelvic floor muscles right before you do that activity.

If you tend to leak urine when you lift something heavy, then try to focus on your pelvic muscles and squeeze *before* you lift it.

Keep squeezing as you lift and remember to breathe. If you leak when you sneeze, try to "squeeze before you sneeze." You'll only have a few seconds to squeeze when you feel a sneeze coming on, but it's enough time to wake up your pelvic floor muscles. Remember to rest your muscles when they start to fatigue. You don't need bionic pelvic floor muscles.

Key In Door Syndrome

Do you feel like you have to pee more when you are trying to get into your house? Do you feel like you might not make it to the bathroom? Do you struggle with getting the key in the lock even more when this is happening? This is called "Key In Door" syndrome. It's referring to the increased urge you are feeling to urinate. Why does this happen? Sometimes getting closer to your door makes you more anxious. The anxiety increases the pressure in your abdomen and causes your bladder to contract. You may even leak a little urine. This is called urge incontinence. Your bladder contractions may also occur due to irritation or nerve issues. What can you do to avoid leaking?

- Relax! You are going to make it!
- Focus on your breathing. Make sure you are taking deep breaths. Taking short and shallow breaths may make you feel more anxious.
- Try contracting your pelvic floor muscles quickly five to six times. These short contractions help to relax the bladder wall and stimulate the sphincter to buy you some time on the way to the bathroom.
- Distract yourself. Think about something other than your bladder. Focusing on your to-do list or latest sonogram picture will help take your mind off of the fact that the bathroom seems like a mile away.

Holly thought she was strengthening her pelvic floor, but she wasn't. She wasn't able to isolate the correct muscles and instead squeezed her butt and leg muscles. That is why she wasn't seeing any progress despite her efforts. Once Holly was able to identify her pelvic floor muscles, she was able to strengthen them. She found the exercises very difficult and often got discouraged. Despite getting stronger, the exercises became more challenging as her baby grew and put more pressure on her weak pelvic floor muscles. She remembered our "Squeeze Before You Sneeze Advice." She squeezed her pelvic floor muscles before sneezing, coughing, laughing, or exerting herself in any way. She followed up with us postpartum. She was worried she had damaged her muscles during delivery. She hadn't. She maintained the strength she developed during her pregnancy and successfully played in the bouncy house with her older daughter. She happily gave her pads to her grandmother-in-law.

Did you ever think you would know so much about your pelvic floor? We want you to be strong enough to support your abdominal organs. We don't want you to pee on yourself! And these muscles shouldn't be too tight and painful. Now that you know how to isolate and use these muscles, let's put them to good use. Enjoy the next chapter on sex throughout your pregnancy.

CHAPTER 4

Between the Sheets during Your Pregnancy

Not now, honey, I have a headache

Kathy was apprehensive about having sex during her pregnancy. She was 14-weeks pregnant with twins and worried about hurting the babies, along with further injuring her back. She tended to be shy in bed and wasn't comfortable exploring different positions and techniques. Her partner's frequent requests to have sex were more frustrating than tempting. While we were helping her low back pain, she shared her intimacy concerns with us. Little did she know we could help her with that too!

Your "morning sickness" occurs 24 hours a day. Your body is changing and feels out of control. All your energy has been zapped. You are always nauseous and tired. You are mad at your partner for impregnating you and making you feel this way, as he or she enjoys your favorite bottle of pinot noir. The last thing you want to do is have sex. And this is only the first trimester!

Remember that during your pregnancy (and even after), there is a hormonal storm happening in your body. Hormone levels decrease during some weeks and then skyrocket at other times. You may feel great during your first trimester, or you may feel like you just want to crawl in a hole and not talk to anyone for nine months. Every pregnancy is different.

As your pregnancy progresses, finding comfortable sexual positions may be challenging. Trying to feel sexy may be even more challenging, especially while all the focus is on your pending arrival. Along with your hormones, your libido will fluctuate throughout your pregnancy:

First trimester. Because you are feeling tired, nauseated, and emotional during your first trimester, you may feel a drop in the desire to tackle your partner. You may be worried about a potential miscarriage and feel overwhelmed by the sheer joy (or fear) about becoming a mom. You will also be experiencing a large increase in blood volume. While this can be a good thing (engorgement causing heightened sensation) for some, increased blood flow to the genitals creates a feeling of fullness, making intercourse more uncomfortable and irritating to your lady parts.

Second trimester. During the second trimester, your nausea should subside and your energy levels should stabilize. You've come to terms with the fact there is another human being inside of you growing bigger each day. Your estrogen hormones are increasing, along with your genital sensitivity and vaginal lubrication. This may cause a dramatic increase in your sexual desire. Your partner is very happy these days.

Third trimester. In your last trimester, you may be feeling more uncomfortable, fatigued, short of breath, and swollen—all which may make for feeling not very sexy.

Orgasms Will Help My Pregnancy?

Challenging as it may be, sexual intimacy is an important part of connecting with your partner throughout your pregnancy. Sex and orgasms are important, as you contract your pelvic floor muscles while doing the deed. The bedroom sure beats the gym! Contracting these muscles makes them stronger. And you want strong muscles during your pregnancy to support your growing uterus. Working these muscles out keeps them strong and keeps their tone healthy.

Also, according to psychologist and sex therapist Stephanie Buehler, orgasms can be more pleasurable during pregnancy. "There is increased blood flow to the genitals. Also, the pregnant woman produces more of certain hormones, like oxytocin, that can make orgasms especially intense." And evidence suggests that the oxytocin (the so-called love hormone) can cross the placental barrier to your baby. Good news for you *and* your baby!

Is Sex Safe during Pregnancy?

This thought might have crossed your mind: "I shouldn't have sex while I'm pregnant. I might hurt the baby!" In most cases, it's perfectly safe for you to have intercourse while you are pregnant and you will not hurt the baby. The exception: If your doctor has put you on "pelvic rest," no forms of sexual intercourse are allowed.

The baby is happily cushioned in his or her fluid-filled amniotic sac and cannot be harmed by your intimate practices. The strong muscles of the uterus itself also work to cushion and protect the baby. Contrary to what some men fear, regardless of their generous endowment, they aren't going to poke the baby. But we can humor their sweet (but silly) thoughts.

If anything, we want to make sure that *you* are comfortable during sex. Different positions may be more comfortable and safe for you throughout your pregnancy. You want increased blood flow to the pelvic area and pelvic floor muscle contractions during orgasms. This may heighten the sensation of orgasm and keep the pelvic floor muscles healthy—which will be necessary in your pregnancy when these muscles are supporting the weight of your baby (or babies)!

So, unless your doctor or midwife says otherwise, sex is safe during pregnancy. If you are diagnosed with any of the following conditions, please discuss possible restrictions with your provider. You may be put on pelvic rest (more on this soon).

- Placenta previa
- Cervical weakness
- Pre-term labor or contractions
- Ruptured membranes
- Vaginal bleeding
- Risk of vaginal infection
- Risk of STD
- After amniocentesis (no sex for 72 hours)
- After chorionic villus sampling (no sex for two weeks)

Can Orgasms Trigger Premature Labor?

According to the Mayo Clinic, orgasms can cause uterine contractions, but these contractions are different from the contractions you'll feel during labor. Orgasms—with or without intercourse—aren't likely to increase the risk of premature labor or premature birth. Similarly, sex isn't likely to trigger labor even as your due date approaches.

Sexual Positions

Here are some positions that will be more comfortable for you and safer for both you and the baby.

Spooning

If during your pregnancy you've been suffering from "pubic symphysis separation," or "pubic symphysis dysfunction," then certain positions may be very uncomfortable for you. The pubic symphysis refers to the joint in the front of your pelvis. It is composed of cartilage that connects the two halves of your pelvis. For some women during pregnancy, this joint becomes very sensitive. The cartilage is affected by your increasing pregnancy hormones and the joint can get very sore. So the idea of wrapping your legs passionately around your partner may not seem as romantic when you're experiencing this pain.

A position that may be more practical for you is the spooning position. Lie on your side with your knees bent and together and have your partner lie behind you. This position gives you the opportunity to enjoy maximal contact without having to stress your pubic symphysis joint. Remember to lie on your left side which is safer for you and the baby.

Side sex

If you are experiencing back pain and don't want to lie on your back or be upright, you can try side sex. You and your partner can both lie on your sides and face each other. If you don't have pain in the front of your pelvic area, then this would be a good position for you. You can also wrap your top leg around your partner. Again, try lying on your left side, which is safe for you and the baby.

Edge of bed

Trying different positions around on different parts of the bed may be just as fun as trying different positions with your partner. Positions at the edge of the bed may help your back and pelvis feel less discomfort. You can lie on your side, or briefly on your back, and your partner can be off the bed, kneeling if the bed is low or standing. You can have your legs wrapped around your partner or supported on chairs. Or you can bend your knees and rest your legs on your partner's chest or shoulders. Or he or she can support your legs, pelvis, and/or low back with his or her arms. There are lots of ways to experiment. Just be careful to be properly supported so you don't fall off the bed! You and your partner can end up on the floor, but only if you choose to.

Preggie on top

You can enjoy more control of your movement and position by being on top during intercourse. This is an ideal position for g-spot stimulation as well. As you progress in the pregnancy, you may feel more fatigued or off balance in this position. So you may need to change positions more often.

Not Recommended: On All Fours

If you want to prevent diastasis recti (a separation of the abdominal muscles during pregnancy) or have already developed this condition, you should avoid the "doggie style" sex position. (See Chapters 1 and 2 for more on this condition.) You want to minimize the amount of time spent on your hands and knees. You don't want your uterus putting additional strain on the already weakened connective tissue between your separated abdominal muscles.

There are lots of other positions to choose from, so don't feel too bad. And remember, this is only temporary! You can get back to your favorite naughty positions once your little one is out.

Pelvic Rest

Your doctor may have told you to stay on "pelvic rest." It's not "bed rest," so what does it mean? It means you shouldn't do anything that might cause or increase bleeding or uterine contractions. Nothing can be inserted into the vagina. Nothing includes: penises, fingers, toys, or tampons. Absolutely no orgasms! So you shouldn't just avoid vaginal intercourse, but also oral and anal sex. Masturbation and nipple stimulation are also no-no's. Stimulating the breasts triggers the release of oxytocin, which can cause contractions. Semen contains prostaglandins that can soften your cervix in preparation for dilation. You want to avoid that.

It's important to speak with your doctor or midwife regarding what you are allowed to do. Pelvic rest, just like bed rest, can be in stages. Depending on the severity, you may be allowed to do some activities and not others. For example, you may be put on "strict pelvic rest," which means no exercise in addition to no sex. Or you may be allowed to do light exercise. Never assume you can do something. Always check with your doctor or midwife first.

So I Can't Have Intercourse. What about Outercourse?

Remember, you can't have orgasms when you are on pelvic rest. But that doesn't mean you can't be intimate with your partner. Here are some suggestions on what you can do to help keep the spark alive:

Plan your encounter. As unsexy as that sounds, it may be best for you and your partner to plan how you are going to go about being intimate and safe.

Get creative. You and your partner may be able to maintain your sexual connection with

- Naughty talk
- Sharing fantasies
- Cuddling
- Spooning
- Reading erotica
- Watching sexy videos
- Kissing from head to toe
- Bathing together
- Sensuous massage

Be honest with your partner. Consider bringing him or her to your next prenatal appointment to better understand your restrictions.

Get expert advice. If your pelvic rest limitations are causing tension with your partner, ask your doctor for a referral to a sexual medicine specialist, sexologist, sex therapist, psychiatrist, psychologist, or counselor. You aren't the first woman to struggle with this so let an expert help you explore other ways to be intimate, communicate about sexual needs and limitations, and overcome possible communication barriers.

Once Kathy decided to try some different positions, she and her partner had sex on their sides. She did not have back pain in this position. They found it worked well when facing each other and when he was behind her, as long as they used a lot of pillows for support. We explained that her babies were protected by amniotic fluid in an amniotic sac and strong uterine muscles.

A thick mucus plug sealed the cervix. The penis would never come in contact with the babies during sex. Knowing this helped her relax and enjoy it. She regretted waiting so long, as she found her orgasms to be the strongest she had ever had. And her back pain had become just a "discomfort." Our patient was happy (and her husband sent us flowers).

You're lucky if this chapter pertained to you and you're having fun in bed. For those not having so much fun in bed while bedridden, the next chapter is for you.

CHAPTER 5

Bed Rest: Survival Tips

I no longer want breakfast in bed

Bed rest is one of the most widely used interventions in obstetrics, with as many as 95 percent of obstetricians prescribing it to their patients. Approximately 18 percent of pregnant women are placed on activity restriction at some time during their pregnancy. Doctors may prescribe bed rest if women have contractions before 37 weeks, experience vaginal bleeding, have high blood pressure, have a history of preterm labor, show a low placenta via ultrasound, are carrying multiple babies, or if the fetus isn't growing as expected.

NASA studies have shown that immobility during bed rest is physically devastating. And their studies weren't even conducted on women, let alone pregnant ones! Researchers have shown the negative effects on your muscles, bones, heart, and lungs with extensive inactivity, as well as weight loss, back pain, disrupted sleep cycles, slower digestion, and a slower postpartum recovery. Degeneration of your body begins within 48 hours of being bedridden. The challenges of taking care of a newborn baby/babies just became that much harder. Some bedridden moms tell us they barely have enough strength to hold their babies once they arrive.

While the research doesn't always support bed rest, many of our patients have benefited from it. All we want is for you to have a healthy pregnancy. If your doctor or midwife suggests it, of course you can discuss the pros and cons, but don't fight it. Your provider only wants what is best for you and your baby.

Alli was told she had an insufficient cervix early in her pregnancy and needed to limit her activity. Her condition worsened and she was put on strict bed rest at 24 weeks. Around 10 weeks later, she was given medical clearance to begin walking. She was anxious to finally buy some items for her baby and walked through a mall "as slow as a snail" for an hour. She went into labor and delivered her premature baby that night via C-section. Despite how weak she felt, she was so happy she complied with her bed rest restrictions, as she doesn't think her baby would have survived when it was just 1 pound at the beginning of her bed rest.

We're glad she listened too!

Who Is on Bed Rest?

There are several conditions that may put you in the category of having a high-risk pregnancy, though not all will lead to bed rest.

- Young or "old" maternal age: Teenager or 35 and older
- Lifestyle choices: use of cigarettes, alcohol, or drugs
- Medical obstetric history: Three or more miscarriages, previous pregnancies resulting in low birth weight babies or preterm births
- Previous pregnancy complications: placenta previa, cervical incompetence, preterm labor, and intrauterine growth retardation (baby is too small)
- Medical conditions in mom: diabetes, high blood pressure, cancer, epilepsy, HIV, sexually transmitted diseases, hepatitis, asthma, heart condition, or autoimmune diseases
- Medical conditions of baby: Down syndrome, heart, lung, or kidney problems
- Carrying multiples: twins or more

If you have not been labeled "high risk," but you are concerned that you are experiencing one or more of the conditions listed above, please discuss this with your doctor or midwife.

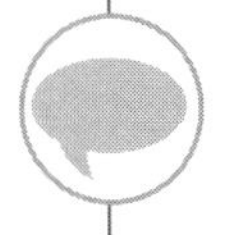

From Jill: Having had two children at 34 and 37, I had more ultrasounds, tests, and fetal monitoring sessions during my second pregnancy. I disputed my high-risk status and questioned the necessity of these procedures simply because I was over 35 years old. In the end, I accepted my old age and never stood up the radiology technicians for my weekly baby photo shoots.

What Is Bed Rest?

With so many different definitions of bed rest, "activity restriction" is a term commonly used in medical literature and research.

Most women are able to be on bed rest at home, although some women need to be hospitalized to allow for close medical monitoring.

If you've been prescribed bed rest, clarify the extent of it. What level of restriction are you on and what are the exact activity restrictions? Some women on bed rest are allowed to sit on a couch, work in their home office, and eat with their families at the table but are not allowed to exercise, have sexual intercourse, or lift anything heavier than a laundry basket.

If your doctor or midwife hasn't given you strict instructions, please inquire. Can you bathe yourself, get up to use the bathroom, prepare meals, drive, work at home, exercise in bed, have sexual intercourse, sleep in a chair? Sidelines National Support Network, a nonprofit organization dedicated to supporting women and their families experiencing complicated pregnancies and premature births, has created a checklist for you to discuss with your doctor or midwife.

What is Bed Rest? Checklist

Date: ______________________

What can I do right now?

Activity level

☐ Maintain a normal activity level
☐ Slightly decrease activity level
☐ Greatly decrease activity level

Working outside the home

☐ Maintain my full-time job
☐ Work part-time ______ hours
☐ Work in my home ______ hours
☐ Stop work completely

Why: ______________________

Working inside the home

☐ Decrease housework including:
  ☐ Heavy lifting (laundry, vacuum)
  ☐ Preparing meals (standing on feet for a prolonged period of time)
  ☐ Other: ______________________

____

Why: ______________________

____

____

____

☐ May use laptop or bedside computer
☐ May sit at computer/desk

Child care

☐ Care for other children as usual
☐ No lifting children
☐ Have caretaker watch active toddler/children

Why: ______________________

____

____

____

Outside stress influences

- ☐ Visitors in home okay? Duration of visits? ______________________________ ______________________________
- ☐ Restriction on types of movies, books (i.e. violent or stress producing)?

Mobility

- ☐ Continue normal mobility
- ☐ Limit mobility (sit down frequently)
- ☐ Lie down each day ______ hours
- ☐ Recline all day (propped up)
- ☐ Lie down flat all day (on side?)
- ☐ May climb stairs _____ times per day
- ☐ May take a shower/wash hair
  Time limit _______
  Times per week _______
- ☐ May take bath/wash hair
- ☐ May eat lying down
- ☐ May eat sitting up
- ☐ May eat sitting at table

Why: ______________________________ ______________________________

Driving

- ☐ May drive a car
  - ☐ As needed.
- ☐ May be a passenger in a car; Frequency: ______________________________
- ☐ May not ride in a car, except to doctor
  - ☐ Sitting up/laying down

Why: ______________________________ ______________________________ ______________________________

Bathroom privileges

- ☐ May use bathroom normally
- ☐ Should actively avoid constipation. How/Treatment: ______________________________ ______________________________
- ☐ Should use bedpan only
- ☐ May use bedside commode

Sexual relations

- ☐ May continue normal sexual relations
- ☐ Should avoid sexual intercourse
- ☐ Should avoid all types of relations which stimulate female orgasm
- ☐ May have occasional sexual relations. How often? ________________

Maintenance of pregnancy

- ☐ Should monitor fetal activity _______ hours each day by hand, counting movements
- ☐ Should monitor for contractions _____ hours daily

Home care

- ☐ Should call perinatal nurse _____ times a week
- ☐ Should use home uterine monitor
- ☐ Should use infusion therapy
  Type: ______________________________
  Purpose: ______________________________ ______________________________
- ☐ Should take medication
  Type: ______________________________
  Times daily/dosage: ________________
  Reason: ______________________________ ______________________________
- ☐ Should take medication
  Type: ______________________________
  Times daily/dosage: ________________
  Reason: ______________________________
- ☐ Should take medication
  Type: ______________________________
  Times daily/dosage: ________________
  Reason: ______________________________ ______________________________
- ☐ Special dietary rules: ________________ ______________________________
  - ☐ Decrease caloric intake
  - ☐ Increase caloric intake

☐ Should take supplements
Type: ______________________
Times daily/dosage: ______________
Reason: ______________________
____
____

What I might expect in the future

☐ May need to self-monitor fetal activity
☐ May need to use a home uterine monitor
☐ May need to take labor-inhibiting drugs
☐ May need to have a cervical stitch put in
☐ May need to stay in hospital
☐ May need to have amniocentesis
☐ May need to have sonograms/ultrasounds
How frequent? ______________
☐ May need to visit OB/GYN more frequently than normal. How frequently?
____
☐ May need to visit a high-risk specialist (Perinatologists)
☐ May need diagnostic test if vaginal fluid is present
When: ______________________
☐ May need to have a blood sugar screening
When: ______________________
☐ May need to have a Non-Stress Test
When: ______________________
May need to have a Stress Test
When: ______________________
☐ May need steroid treatment for baby's lung development
When: ______________________
☐ May need diagnostic test if vaginal fluid is present (AmniSure test) or conventional clinical assessment.

If problems arise

☐ At what point should I contact my OB/GYN? ______________
☐ Which hospital should I go to in case of emergency? ______________
____
☐ Names of Neonatologist/Pediatricians to consult? ______________
____
☐ If needed, where would my baby be hospitalized? ______________
____
____
☐ What is the possibility of a cesarean section? ______________
____
____
☐ additional instructions
____
____
____
____
____

Doctor's Office #: ______________
After Hours #: ______________
Other doctors that might be on call
____
____
____

☐ Other Emergency #: ______________
____
____
____
____

Discuss your Sidelines bed rest checklist with your doctor or midwife. Once cleared to exercise in bed, see the Let's Get Physical section on page 147 for some safe exercises (pending your health care provider's clearance!) that will help you maintain your strength.

Sidelines (www.sidelines.org), established in 1991, is an excellent source of support if you have a high-risk pregnancy. They have helped over 200,000 families through e-mail and phone support.

Is Bed Rest Necessary?

Maybe. What is interesting about bed rest is that despite its prevalence, the literature doesn't equivocally support its effectiveness. Recent literature shows that activity restriction does not prevent preterm labor or infant mortality, even in women carrying multiples. This was studied in 713 women carrying 1,452 babies that were on hospital bed rest. Cochrane reviews of bed rest have been studied and researchers conclude that "therapeutic" bed rest for threatened abortion, hypertension, preeclampsia, preterm birth, multiple gestations, or impaired fetal growth is not supported. Other institutions believe that bed rest eases contractions, reduces the pull on the uterus and resulting pressure on the cervix, lessens the chance of further cervical opening, and lowers your blood pressure.

The Emotional Toll

Being put on bed rest probably sounds like a jail sentence to you. And it is, somewhat. We understand that. Stress, frustration, anxiety, and depressive symptoms are just a few emotions expressed by women on bed rest. Research has shown that the anxiety, depression, and hostility seen in pregnant patients on bed rest may not be caused by the actual bed rest, but by other factors such as their pregnancy in jeopardy, financial stress, or medical complications. The depression lessens as the pregnancy progresses and is lowest after delivery.

While we can help you physically survive bed rest, we consulted with an expert to help you with the emotional aspect. Dr. Sabrina Khan, Clinical Assistant Professor at New York University School of Medicine and psychiatrist specializing in reproductive psychiatry/women's mental health, offers the following:

Are You Depressed?

While pregnancy can be a special time for women, for some it can be extremely difficult physically, emotionally, or both. Unfortunately, many women suffering from depression or anxiety are afraid to talk about their distressing symptoms, or they experience guilt for feeling this way. As a result, their illness is undiagnosed and untreated.

At least 14.5 percent of women suffer from perinatal depression, making it the most common, but often missed, complication of pregnancy.

But it doesn't have to be.

Are You at Risk?

Depression in pregnancy can happen to anyone. It is not uncommon for a woman with no prior history of psychiatric illness to develop new onset depression or anxiety while pregnant or postpartum. Risk factors for perinatal depression include a past history of depression, a family history of depression, recent discontinuation of an antidepressant, medical or obstetrical complications, history of trauma or abuse, history of drug or alcohol abuse, a major stressful life event, and lack of support.

What to Watch for:

Some of the physical symptoms of major depression—a change in appetite, fatigue or loss of energy, change in sleep—can be easily mistaken as common symptoms of pregnancy. In addition to these, depression is marked by the following symptoms for at least two weeks.

- Depressed or irritable mood, most of the day, nearly every day
- Decreased interest or pleasure in most activities
- Feelings of guilt or worthlessness
- Difficulty concentrating or indecisiveness
- Thoughts of death or suicide

While anxiety is another distressing symptom commonly experienced during a depressive episode, it can also be a comorbid disorder and therefore should be evaluated.

An effective screening tool is the Edinburgh Postnatal Depression Scale (EPDS), which follows. Talk to your health care provider now about how you are feeling if you score 10 or greater, or have thoughts of death or suicide.

Edinburgh Postnatal Depression Scale

Check the answer that comes closest to how you have felt in the past seven days, not just how you feel today.

1. I have been able to laugh and see the funny side of things.
    - o As much as I always could
    - o Not quite so much now

- o Definitely not so much now
- o Not at all

2. I have looked forward with enjoyment to things.
   - o As much as I ever did
   - o Rather less than I used to
   - o Definitely less than I used to
   - o Hardly at all
3. I have blamed myself unnecessarily when things went wrong.
   - o Yes, most of the time
   - o Yes, some of the time
   - o Not very often
   - o No, never
4. I have been anxious or worried for no good reason.
   - o No, not at all
   - o Hardly ever
   - o Yes, sometimes
   - o Yes, very often
5. I have felt scared or panicky for no very good reason.
   - o Yes, quite a lot
   - o Yes, sometimes
   - o No, not much
   - o No, not at all
6. Things have been getting on top of me.
   - o Yes, most of the time I haven't been able to cope at all
   - o Yes, sometimes I haven't been coping as well as usual
   - o No, most of the time I have coped quite well
   - o No, I have been coping as well as ever

7. I have been so unhappy that I have had difficulty sleeping.
    - o Yes, most of the time
    - o Yes, sometimes
    - o Not very often
    - o No, not at all
8. I have felt sad or miserable.
    - o Yes, most of the time
    - o Yes, quite often
    - o Not very often
    - o No, not at all
9. I have been so unhappy that I have been crying.
    - o Yes, most of the time
    - o Yes, quite often
    - o Only occasionally
    - o No, never
10. The thought of harming myself has occurred to me.
    - o Yes, quite often
    - o Sometimes
    - o Hardly ever
    - o Never

Scoring

Questions 1, 2, & 4 (without an *) Are scored 0, 1, 2 or 3 with top box scored as 0 and the bottom box scored as 3.

Questions 3, 5–10 (marked without an *) Are reverse scored, with the top box scored as a 3 and the bottom box scored as 0.

Maximum score: 30

Possible Depression: 10 or greater

Always look at item 10 (suicidal thoughts)

Why Is Diagnosis So Important?

Your well-being matters, for you and for your family. Major depression hurts, and can impact your pregnancy. Left untreated, it can result in poor self-care/prenatal care; self-medication with tobacco, alcohol, or drugs; postpartum depression; and sadly, in very serious cases, suicide. The biggest predictor of postpartum depression is antenatal depression.

Perinatal depression has been associated with preterm birth and low birth weight.

Are Antidepressants Safe?

Depending on the severity of symptoms, treatment with psychotherapy alone or with an antidepressant can help you feel yourself again.

In 2009, after a thorough review of the research, the American College of Obstetrics and Gynecology and the American Psychiatric Association published guidelines for the treatment of perinatal depression. The potential adverse effects of medication on the fetus must always be measured against the effects of untreated maternal illness. While mild to moderate depression may be treated with psychotherapy alone, antidepressant treatment is indicated in severe depression. Fortunately, most antidepressants are also compatible with breastfeeding.

More recently in 2013, Grigoriadis et al. published a meta-analysis of studies looking at antidepressant treatment in pregnancy and also concluded that antidepressants do not appear to be associated with an increased risk of congenital malformations, though findings are inconsistent due to limitations in the studies. In individual studies that have noted an increase in the risk of cardiovascular malformations, the absolute risk is quite small.

Byatt et al. published a review of the literature regarding antidepressant use in pregnancy, with similar conclusions. They also discuss the possible risk of postnatal adaptation syndrome (marked by irritability, abnormal crying, tremor, lethargy, hypoactivity, decreased feeding, or respiratory distress in the newborn) in up to 30 percent of exposed babies. However, this would not be a reason to discontinue treatment late in pregnancy, as the symptoms are self-limited. A detailed discussion of these findings is beyond the scope of this book, but consult your healthcare provider about the benefits versus risks of antidepressant treatment. Unfortunately, there is no such thing as no exposure; lack of treatment for mom can leave the baby exposed to the effects of depression and anxiety. Studies have shown that severe stress in pregnancy can impact the neurodevelopment of the baby; severe prenatal stress and anxiety has been associated with an increased risk for emotional and behavioral issues in the child.

There Is Hope

Tell your doctor or midwife how you feel; they may provide treatment for you or refer you to a psychiatrist who can further evaluate your symptoms. We can't ever overestimate the importance of a mom who is well.

Let's Get Physical

Once approved by your doctor or midwife, here are some exercises that can be done in bed. Share this list of exercises with your health care provider and have him or her specifically clear you for each one. This will avoid any confusion or miscommunication. While we want you to be as strong as you can be while bedridden, the health of you and your baby is most important. Please make sure to let your provider know if you experience any uterine contractions, pain, bleeding or amniotic fluid loss. Remember, these exercises are designed to lessen the effects of bed rest. You shouldn't be exerting yourself too much. This isn't a Jillian Michaels workout. There are several reasons we want you to exercise.

Bed Rest Strategies for Keeping Sane

- **Organizing unit**. Why not make your time on bed rest a little easier with help from an organizing unit? Keep your corner tidy with a simple box or a special tray. This will help you keep your TV and DVD remotes, phone, and other important accessories in an easy-to-access spot. You don't have time to hunt for your phone—oh yeah, you do, but you don't want to. Laptop, books, games, art projects, music, knitting, plastic utensils, and paper plates (cut yourself some slack on being green for once).
- **Lap desk**. Use a lap desk for reading, writing, eating, crafts, puzzles, and games. It is an essential item on your bed rest shopping list.
- **Radio or baby monitor**. If you're on strict bed rest—no getting up at all (unless you're using the restroom, and even that only under accompaniment)—a two-way radio or baby monitor can be essential. Both will help you communicate easily with people in other rooms.

1. Exercise will help break up the boredom and monotony of your bed rest restriction.
2. Exercise will give you a sense of empowerment. You may be confined to your bed, but you can still make your muscles stronger to prepare for your little one's arrival.
3. Exercise will improve your circulation so blood doesn't pool.
4. Exercise will decrease your muscle and joint stiffness from lying in bed so long.
5. Exercise is something you can do with your family or friends.

For all of the following exercises, start slow. Perform a set of 10 repetitions and see how you feel. If you feel good, do another set of 10. You can perform the exercise using just one side (left or right arm/leg) or you can do both limbs at the same time. Listen to your body. And keep breathing throughout the exercises!

Upper Body

Keeping your upper body strong is important, as you need the strength to hold and care for your newborn. (Not to mention any other kids you already have that weigh significantly more). You (or your helpful partner) can take a piece of resistance band and tie it to the leg of your bed while you are lying down. Feel free to prop yourself up with pillows to make yourself as comfortable as possible.

Muscle group: biceps

Benefits: Your biceps are the muscles on the front of your upper arm. You use these muscles to gently lower your baby into a crib or pick up things such as babies, boxes, laundry baskets, your partner's clothes off the floor, and so on.

Exercise:

- Tie a resistance band to the leg of your bed. Hold the other end of the resistance band in your right hand.
- Bend and straighten your elbow. Try to keep your elbow in the same spot while you are bending your arm.

You can hold the band with more or less resistance to vary the intensity of the exercise. So if it feels too difficult, give yourself more slack in the band or try a band with less resistance.

You can also do this exercise with a water bottle, light dumbbell, or other drink bottle. You can adjust the weight by filling or emptying the bottle with more or less fluid.

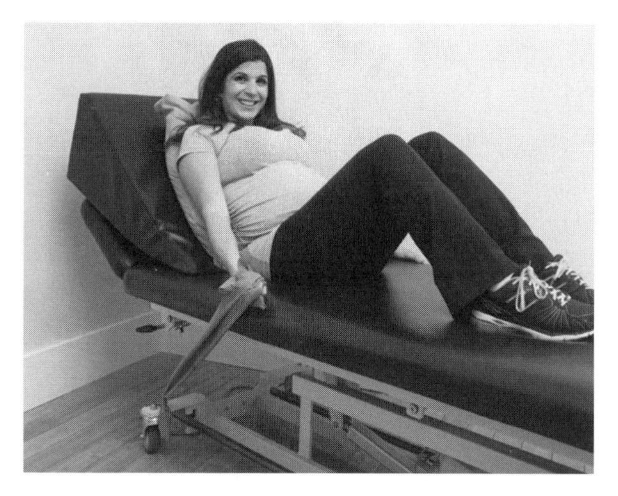
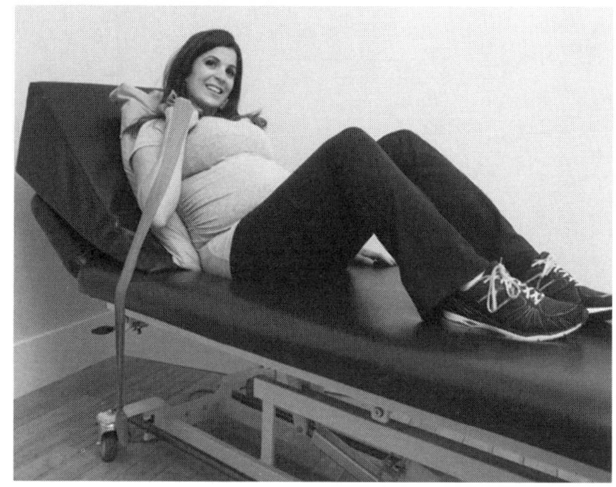

Biceps strengthening (bicep curls) with resistance band

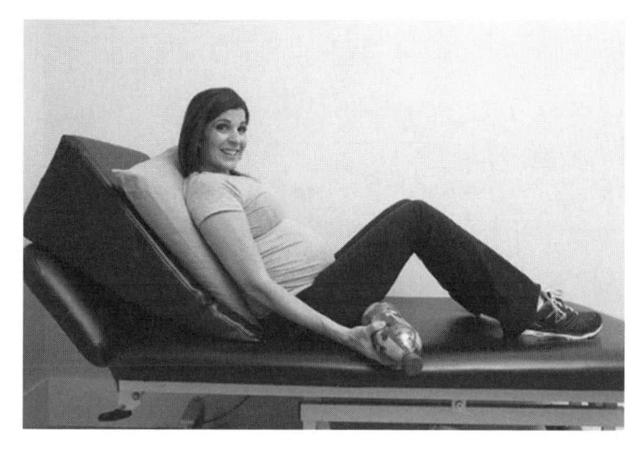
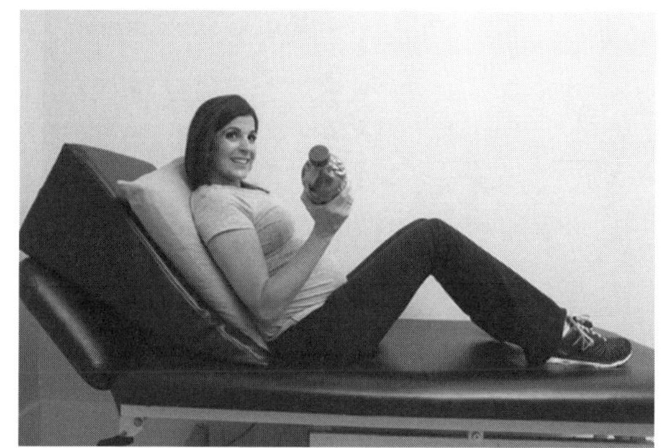

Biceps strengthening (bicep curls) with weight

Muscle group: triceps

Benefits: Now that you have worked out the muscles in the front of your upper arm, we need to target the muscles in the back of your upper arm, your triceps. This muscle helps you push yourself up from a chair or low surface when you stand up. Yes, you will eventually be able to get out of bed.

Exercise:

- Keep the resistance band tied to the leg of the bed.
- Hold the other end of the band in your right hand and bring your hand behind your head for the starting position. Your elbow should be pointing up toward the ceiling.
- Now, raise your hand toward the ceiling without moving your elbow. Imagine you are punching the ceiling with your fist.

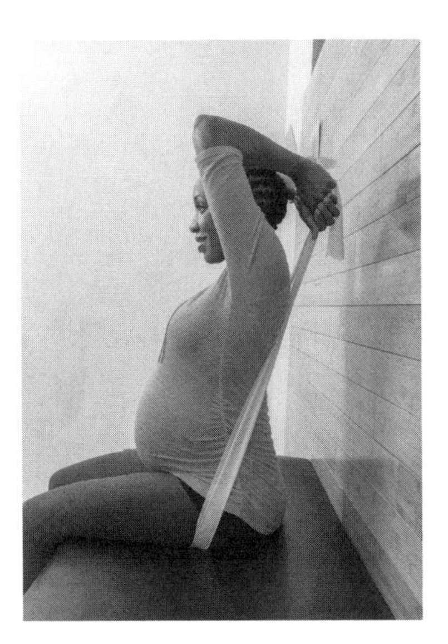
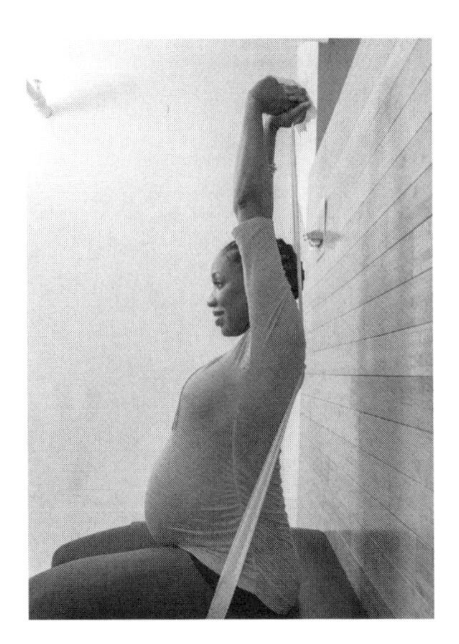

Tricep strengthening (overhead tricep extension)

Muscle group: deltoids

Benefits: Your deltoids are located on the rounded part of your shoulders and top of your outer arms. You use these muscles when you reach for something overhead in your closet, drive, put your hair in a ponytail, or lift your little one in the air and pretend she is an airplane.

Exercise:

- Start with your hands at shoulder level.
- Raise your arm up toward the ceiling. This is different from your triceps exercises because you are moving your whole arm toward the ceiling instead of just your fist and forearm.
- Again, keep breathing.

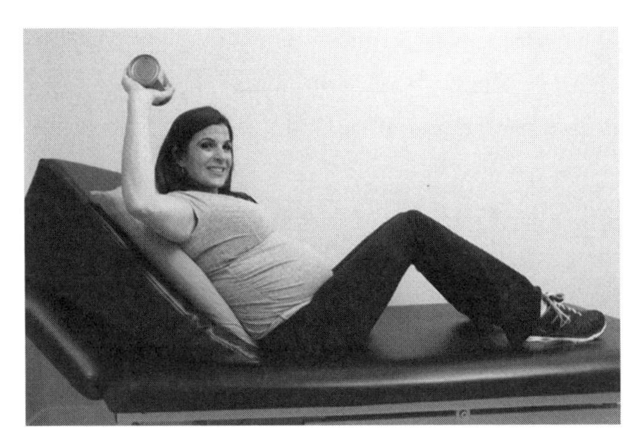
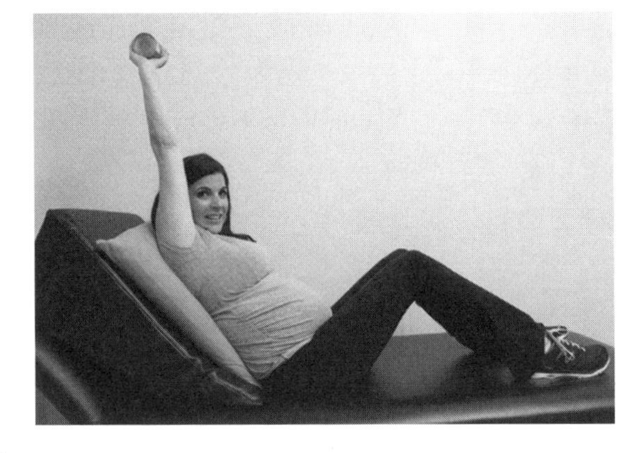

Deltoid strengthening (shoulder presses) with weight

Exercise, with a resistance band:

- Bend your knees and keep your back propped up with pillows. Place the resistance band under your thighs.
- Hold the ends in each hand at shoulder level.
- Lift both of your hands up toward the ceiling.

Don't strain to do the exercise. If the resistance band is too heavy, use a thinner/easier band.

You can also work different muscle fibers of the deltoids by lying on your side.

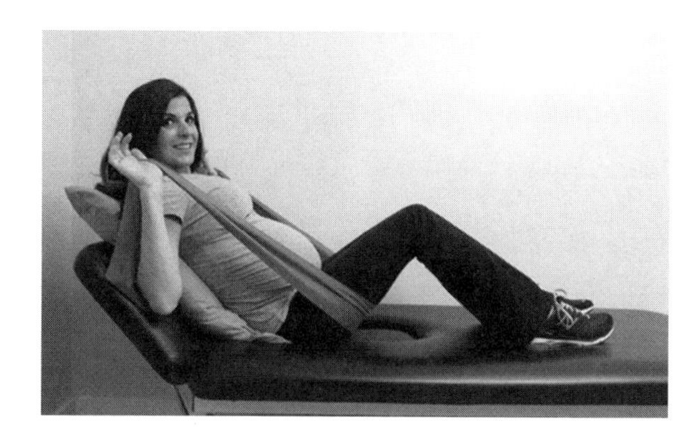

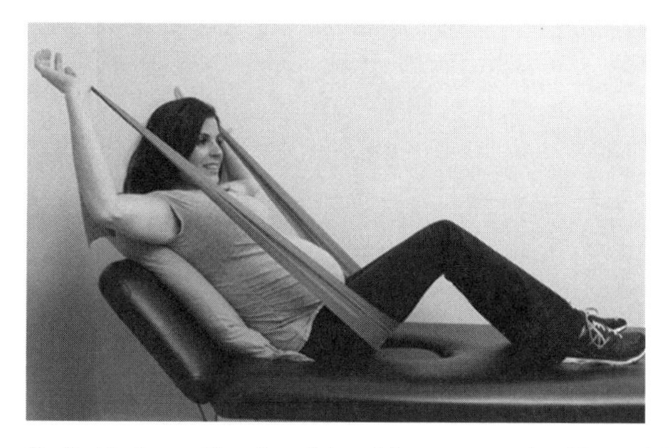

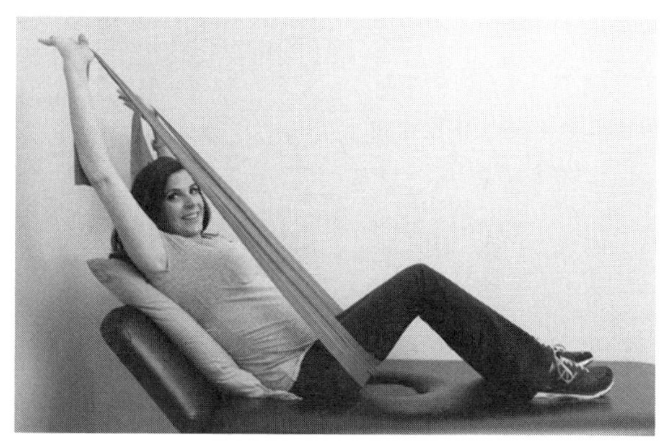

Deltoid strengthening (shoulder presses) with resistance band

Exercise:

- Lie on your side.
- Keep your elbow straight and lift your arm straight up toward the ceiling in an arc.

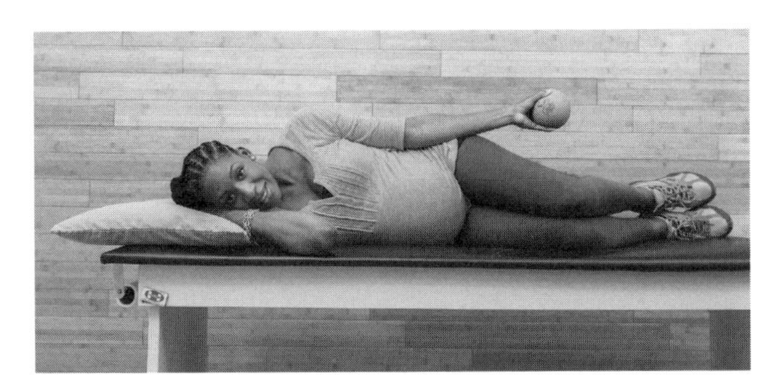

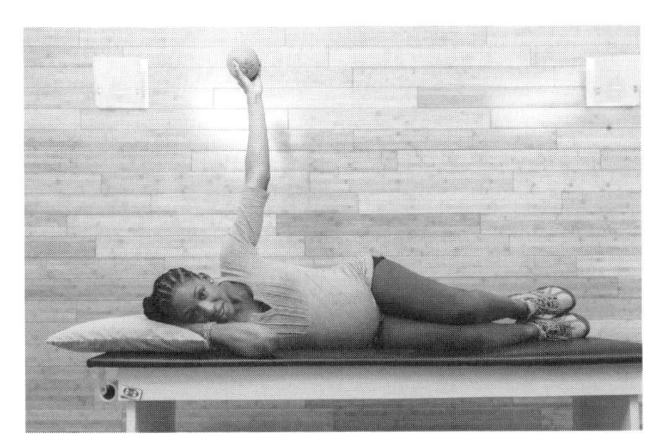

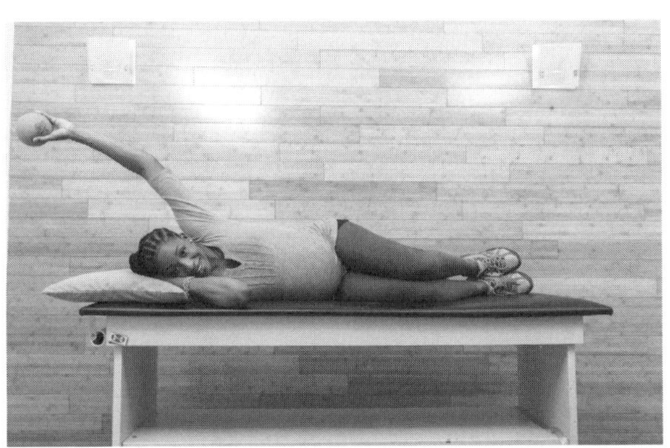

Deltoid strengthening (arcs)

Muscle group: pectoralis major/minor

Benefits: Your "pecs" are your chest muscles. You may feel that you are slouching more while you are on bed rest. Or you may feel as though your breasts are heavy and making your chest feel tight. These muscles help you to pick up your little one and hold him or her close as during nursing or feeding, lift bags of groceries, or hold two children at the same time. You strengthen these muscles by squeezing your arms together in front of you.

Exercise:

- Hold a hand weight in each hand and extend your arms out to your sides. You can bend your elbows or keep them straight.
- Bring your hands together in front of you.
- Remember to squeeze the muscles as you bring your hands together.

Always keep breathing.

You can adjust the weight by emptying or filling the water bottles.

Stretch: You can also stretch these muscles by rolling your shoulders *back* in a circular motion while propped up in bed. Think about squeezing your shoulder blades together and down. You don't need to roll them forward, as your shoulders have most likely already creeped forward into this hunched position.

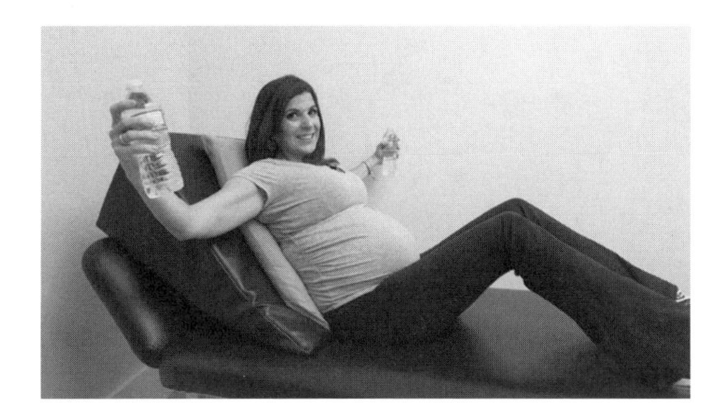

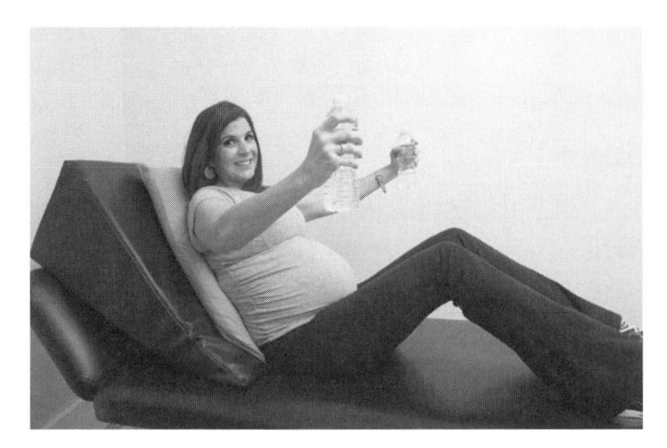

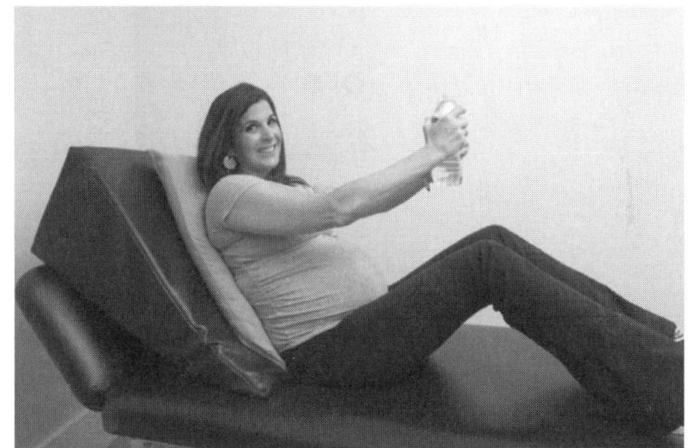

Pectoral (chest muscle) strengthening (chest squeezes)

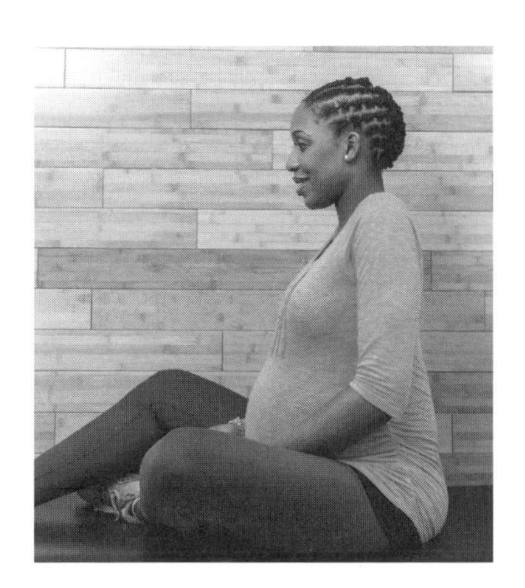

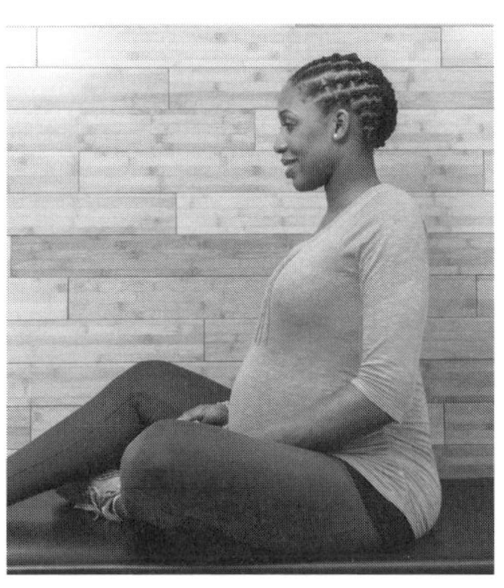

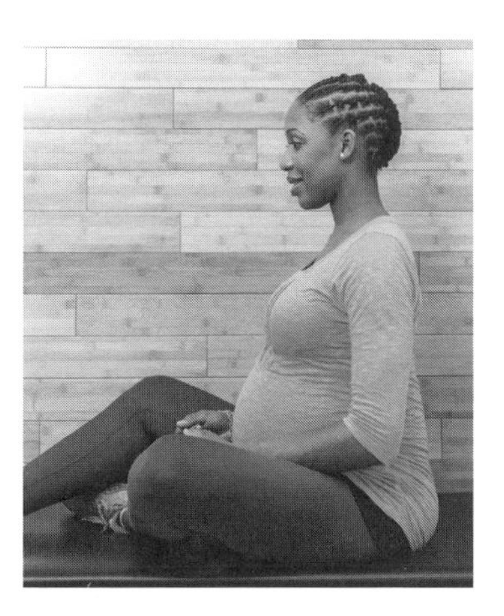

Shoulder circles: Dynamic shoulder stretching

Stretch: Another way to stretch these muscles is by bringing your arms out to the side while you are lying down. Bend your elbows so that your elbows as well as your shoulders are at 90 degree angles. Make sure your arms are flat against the bed. Feel the stretch in the front of your chest and shoulders.

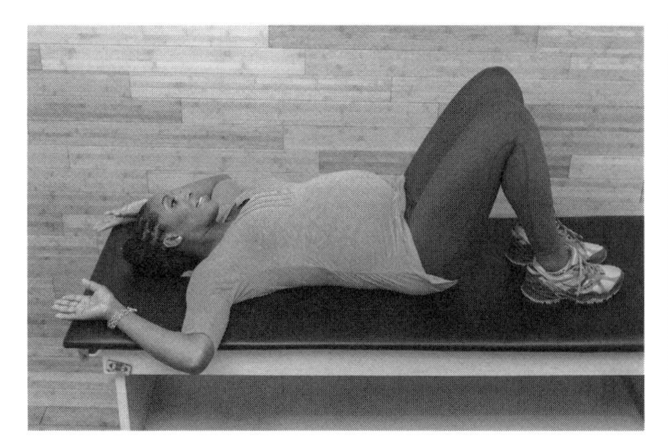
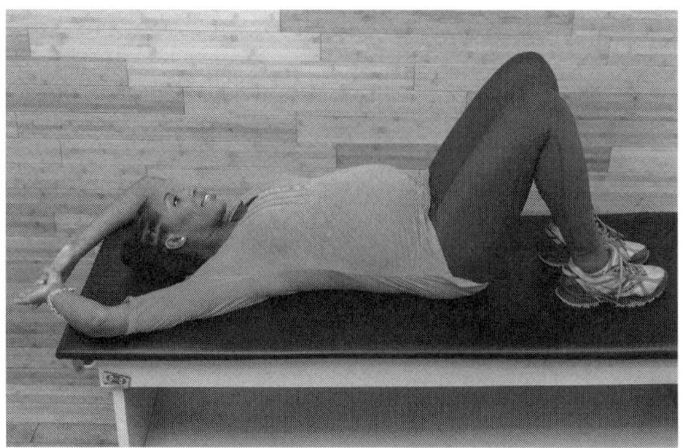

Chest muscle stretch

Core

Muscle group: abdominals

Benefits: This stretch will keep your abdomen and hips mobile, helping you to roll onto your side, when you're ready to get out of bed. And when that day comes, we want you to be ready!

Stretch, trunk roll:

- Lie on your back (propped up with pillows), with your knees bent and feet flat.
- Move your knees to the right of your body.
- Let your body relax into this position for 30 seconds. You should feel a gentle stretch along the sides of your abdomen.
- Switch to the left side and hold for 30 seconds.
- Depending on your baby's orientation, one side may feel tighter than the other.
- Alternate until you've done five stretches on each side.

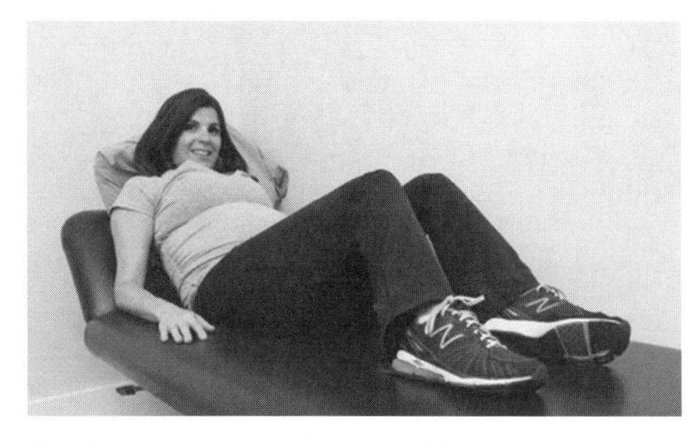
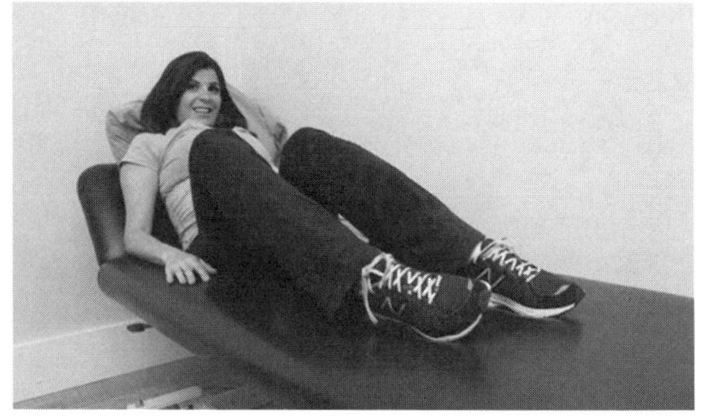

Trunk strengthening (trunk rolls)

Lower Body

Muscle groups: anterior tibialis and gastrocnemius

Benefits: These are your shin and calf muscles. These muscles, in the front and back of your lower legs, hold up your feet so you don't trip over your toes. They also help with ankle stability and balance. Plus, they help with the kicking motion, if you need to clear a path through too many toys or your partner isn't helping you with chores. Strong calves enable you to go up onto your tippy-toes to reach the high shelf where you are hiding things from your partner or child.

When you walk, your calf muscles pump blood out of your legs and up toward your heart. When you are on bed rest and unable to walk, the blood can pool in your calves and form a clot. The clot can travel throughout your body and can get stuck in a small blood vessel. You definitely don't want this is to happen, so let's get those calves pumping.

Exercise: Ankle pumps are an easy way to keep blood pumping through your calves. Do these throughout the day when confined to bed.

Move the top of your foot toward your shin and then away from it to strengthen these muscles and keep your ankles mobile. You can do this exercise with your knees bent or straight.

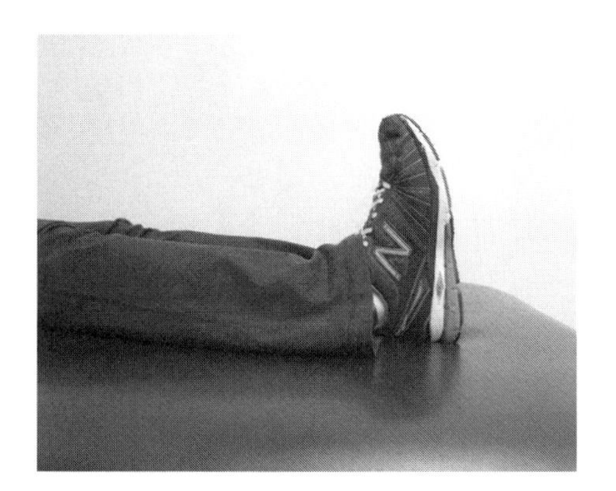
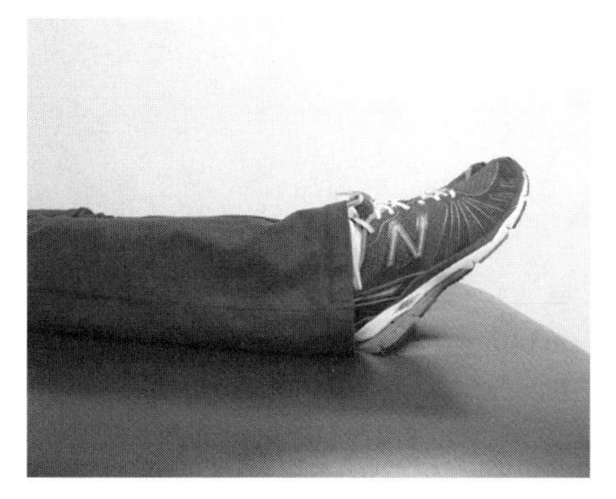

Anterior tibialis and gastrocnemius strengthening (ankle pumps)

Muscle groups: gluteus maximus and hamstrings

Benefits: Your gluteus maximus muscles are your butt muscles and will someday be the strongest muscles in your body. Your hamstrings are the long muscles behind your thighs that begin at your pelvis and end just below your knees. Both of these muscle groups can get weak during pregnancy when your pelvis tilts forward with your growing bump. Throw bed rest into the picture and these muscles never get a workout.

Having a strong bum and legs help you move around in bed when you need to change positions, climb stairs, walk, get out of a chair, and stand upright. If you are using a bed pan during your bed rest, having strong muscles will make it easier to lift your hips when you need to use it. Plus, a strong butt gives you sturdy hips to hold your baby on your side.

Exercise: A very easy way you can work your gluteus maximus is by squeezing your butt cheeks together. Keep your knees straight for this one. (You don't need a picture for this exercise, just squeeze your butt muscles.)

Hold the contraction for 10 seconds, rest, and repeat 10 times.

If this gets too easy, practice some bridges.

Exercise:

- Bend both of your knees. Feet are flat and hip-width apart.
- Lift your butt off the bed a couple of inches.
- Tighten your butt as you do this and hold the position for three seconds.

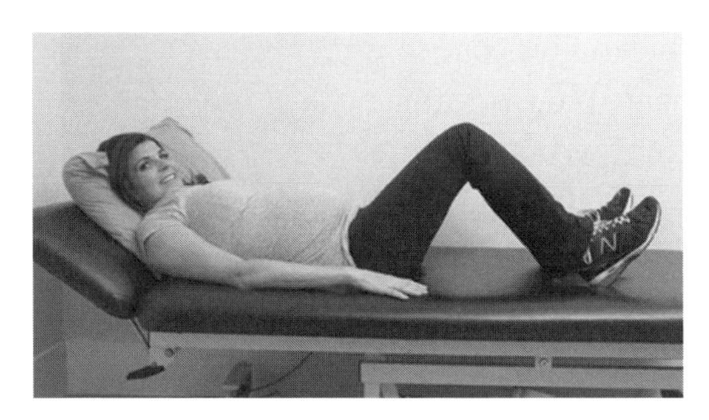

Hamstring strengthening

Refer to pages 3 to 4 for pictures of bridging.

Exercise:

- To strengthen your hamstrings, keep your knees bent and dig your heels into the bed. Make sure to keep your toes up and your heels down.

Remember to breathe. *Never hold your breath.*

Muscle groups: gluteus medius and obturator internus (hip rotators)

Benefits: The gluteus medius muscles are located on the side of your hips. These muscles help lift your leg out to the side and stabilize your pelvis when you walk. Each time you swing your left leg forward, your right gluteus medius contracts so your pelvis doesn't drop and you don't fall over. These muscles also kick in when you stand on one leg to put your pants on, tie a shoe lace, do the hokey pokey, or perform any other activity you do while standing on one leg.

The hip rotators turn your legs outward. You use this motion when you are getting out of a car.

Exercise:

- To strengthen your hip rotators, lie on your side and bend both knees.
- Separate your knees by turning the top leg outward. Picture how a clam shell opens. Make sure you keep your ankles together.

You can also perform this exercise by tying a resistance band around your thighs and separating your knees against the resistance of the band.

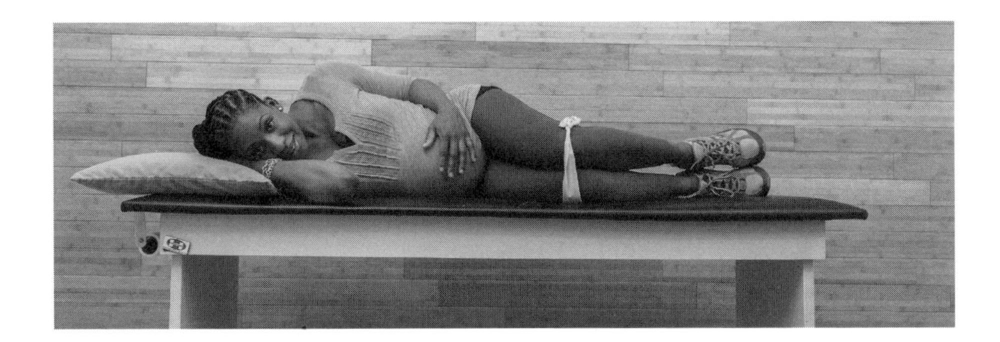

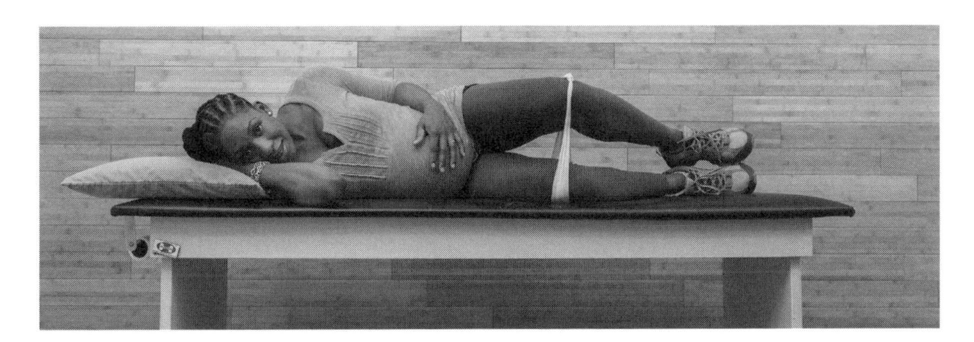

Clam shell exercise using a resistance band

Exercise:

- To strengthen your gluteus medius, stay in this position (on your side). You can slide the resistance band down so it's around your ankles.
- Straighten your legs and make sure your body is in as much of a straight line as possible.
- Slowly lift your top leg until you feel your outer hip muscles working. DO NOT do this if you have pelvic pain, as it could exacerbate your symptoms.
- Lift the top leg toward the ceiling and contract the muscles on the side of your hip.

Muscle group: quadriceps (quads)

Benefits: The quadriceps are located in the front of your thigh and can't be ignored while on bed rest. These muscles help you control a squat position, like when you are bending down to pick up your baby or hovering over a public toilet seat. You need these muscles to walk and get up and down the stairs.

Exercise:

- You can strengthen them by sitting at the edge of your bed and straightening your right leg by lifting your foot.
- Straighten your knee as much as you can and make sure to tighten your quad muscle.

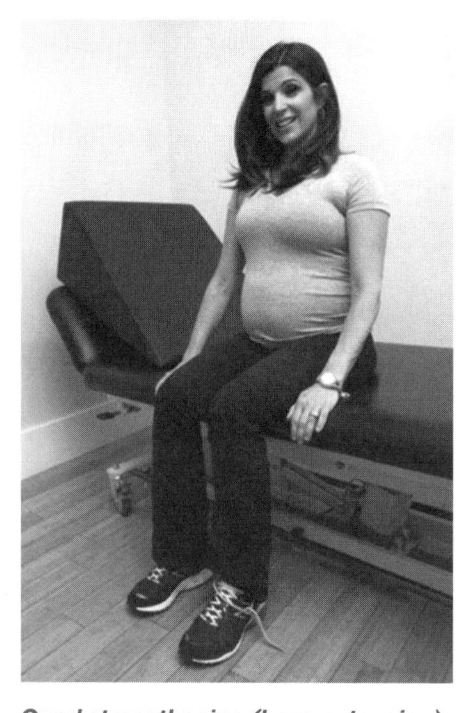

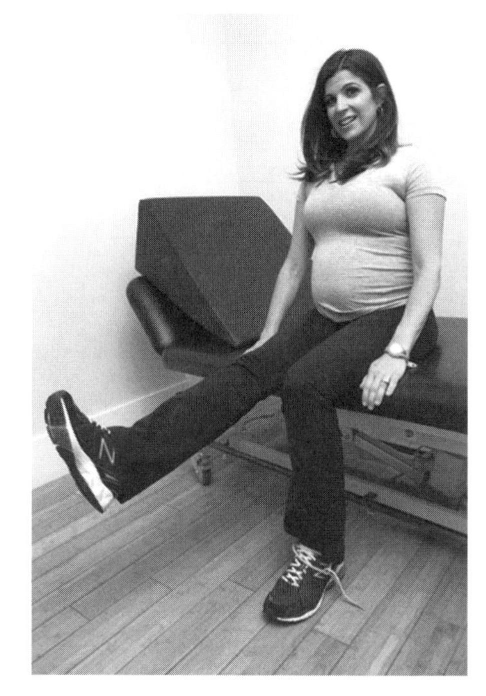

Quad strengthening (knee extension)

You can also do this exercise using a resistance band tied around your ankles.

Lauren said, "It took me much longer to recover after my second C-section. I wasn't on bed rest during my first pregnancy, so it was a different experience. I don't know if it was because I did nothing for two and a half months or because it was my second baby. I believe it was because my muscles weren't used in so long. After my first daughter was born, I was up and about in one to two weeks. It took much longer for sure with my second. I wouldn't

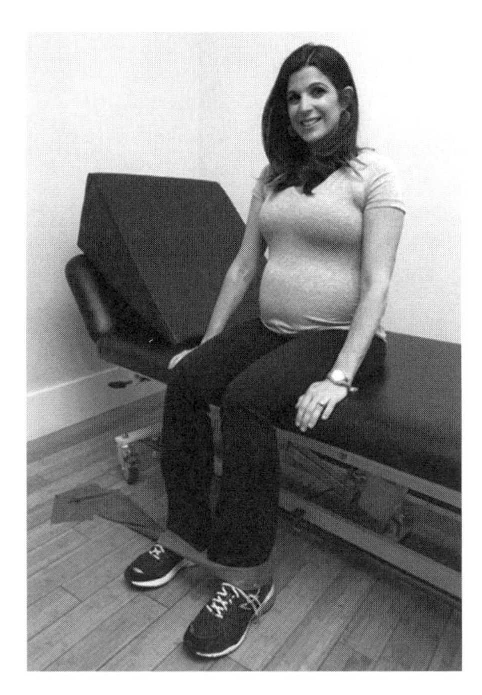
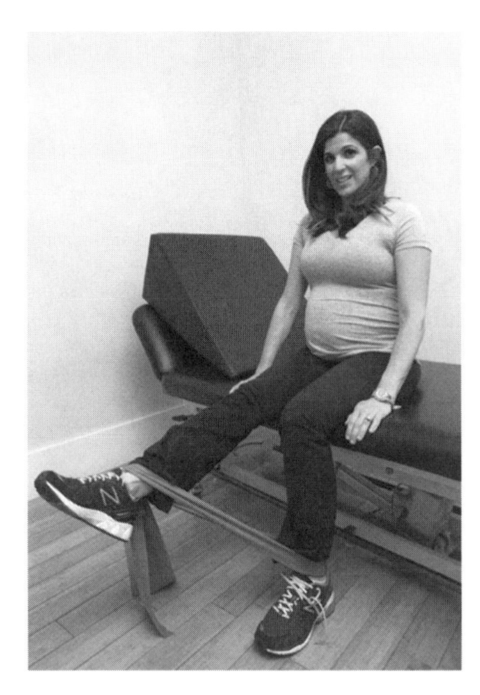

Quad strengthening (knee extension with resistance band)

change how I did things at all. My baby's health was much more important to me than my fitness. I made sure I continued to eat healthy so that helped. I think if I was a person who wasn't physically fit originally the experience and recovery would be completely different."

Soon you will be out of bed and enjoying your little one(s). The next chapter will help with labor and delivery, if you don't already have a C-section planned.

CHAPTER 6

Planning for Labor and Delivery

I need to stretch my what??

Grab the hospital bag! Where are the car keys?? You're in labor! You're huffing and puffing your way through your contractions and you're wondering if you'll be huffing for several minutes, hours, or days. You're focused on having a smooth labor and delivery and you have all your labor-related paraphernalia in tow. We want your birthing experience to be positive, so let's go over several things you can do to get prepared for your little one's grand entrance.

True Labor vs. False Labor

Don't grab that hospital bag just yet. You may not actually be in labor. Before "true" labor begins, you might have "false" labor pains, also known as Braxton Hicks contractions. According to the Cleveland Clinic, these irregular uterine contractions are perfectly normal and might start to occur from your fourth month of pregnancy. They are your body's way of getting ready for the "real thing."

Braxton Hicks (false labor) contractions:

- Feel like tightening in the abdomen that comes and goes.
- Do not get closer together.
- Do not increase in how long they last.
- Do not increase in how often they occur.

- Do not feel stronger over time.
- Often come with a change of position and stop with rest.
- May stop when you walk or rest.
- May stop when you change position.

True contractions:

- Feel different for each woman.
- May feel different from one pregnancy to the next.
- Cause discomfort or a dull ache in your back and lower abdomen.
- Cause pressure in the pelvis.
- May cause pain in your side and thighs.
- May feel like strong menstrual cramps or diarrhea cramps.
- Come at regular intervals and get closer together as time goes on (should last about 30–70 seconds).
- Continue, despite moving or changing positions.

Perineal Massage

Since you will be trying to push a little watermelon out through your vagina, you want to make sure your vagina is ready for the job. During the second stage of labor (that's when you are actively pushing your little one out), you may tear or have an episiotomy. An episiotomy is when your doctor or midwife makes an incision on the perineum and the posterior vaginal wall to help your baby come out.

Episiotomy

There isn't much current evidence justifying the routine use of episiotomy in order to avoid perineal trauma. In fact, the American Congress of Obstetrics and Gynecology in 2006 recommended the *"restricted* use of episiotomies." This means that physicians should only use this technique when it's absolutely necessary for the health and safety of mom and baby. Episiotomies have been linked to severe lacerations in the pelvic floor, from the vagina to the anal sphincter. These lacerations can occur in subsequent births too. With episiotomies, there is more bleeding during delivery, scarring, increased pain, sexual dysfunction, and increased costs. Episiotomies do not prevent postpartum pelvic floor pain or dysfunction.

Please know, in some cases, an episiotomy may actually benefit the mother and the baby. In case of true fetal distress (determined by abnormal changes in heart rate on the fetal monitor) the baby may need to be born immediately. Enlarging the vaginal opening may help facilitate the delivery. An episiotomy can also be beneficial if the baby is particularly large or the mother is unable to push anymore.

The doctors and midwives have read the research. The rate of episiotomy with all vaginal deliveries decreased from 60.9 percent in 1979 to 24.5 percent in 2004. There is a lot of variability in the prevalence of episiotomies around the world. It is highest in Latin America and lower in Europe, with reported rates varying widely from 1 percent in Sweden to 80 percent in Argentina.

Katie wishes her doctors weren't so scissor-happy. She developed painful scar tissue from her episiotomy. Her OB treated her scar tissue by cauterizing the area with silver nitrate. It took six months for the pain to resolve and she needed to sit on ice for several hours after each painful procedure. She wishes she never had an episiotomy, but never discussed other options with her doctor during her prenatal appointments.

You may simply tear during delivery. And that is OK. It is often better to tear than to be cut." What nature separates, nature heals." An episiotomy doesn't shorten the length of your second stage of labor. It doesn't save your pelvic floor muscles. And it doesn't enable you to return to comfortable sex sooner. Research actually shows the opposite.

So how do you avoid the surgical scissors? By stretching and massaging your perineum so that your doctor doesn't have to cut you. This process is called "antenatal perineal massage." Antenatal perineal massage reduces the likelihood of perineal trauma (mainly episiotomies) and the reporting of ongoing perineal pain, according to several studies. One study from 2012 found that there was a reduction in third- and fourth-degree tears with massage of the perineum.

Some research says it helps. Others say it doesn't make a difference. There is no evidence of harm—so give it a shot.

According to the *Journal of Midwifery and Women's Health,* follow these instructions if you wish to use perineal massage:

- Begin four to six weeks before your due date.
- Wash your hands well, and keep your fingernails short. Relax in a private place with your knees bent. Some women like to lean on pillows for back support.
- Lubricate your thumbs and the perineal tissues. Use a lubricant such as vitamin E oil or almond oil, or any vegetable oil used for cooking—like olive oil.You may also try a water-soluble jelly, such as K-Y jelly, or your body's natural vaginal lubricant. Do not use baby oil, mineral oil, or petroleum jelly.
- Place your thumbs about 1 to 1.5 inches inside your vagina. Press down (toward the anus) and to the sides until you feel a slight burning, stretching sensation.
- Hold that position for one or two minutes. With your thumbs, slowly massage the lower half of the vagina using a "U" shaped movement. Concentrate on relaxing your muscles. This is a good time to practice slow, deep breathing techniques.

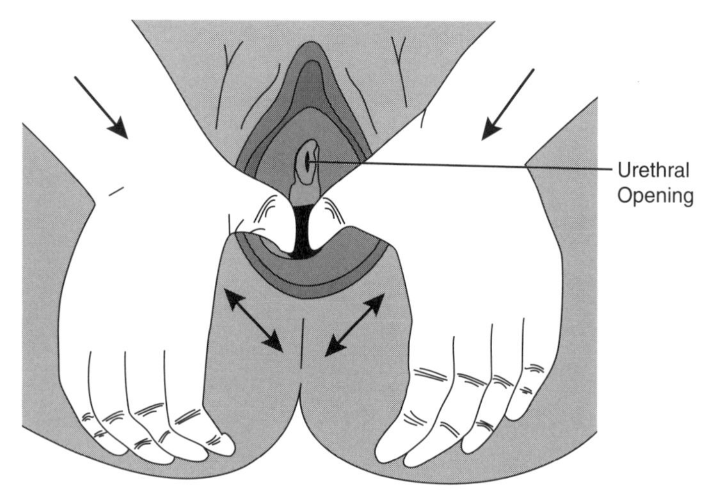

- Massage your perineal area slowly for 10 minutes each day. After one to two weeks, you should notice more stretchiness and less burning in your perineum.

Partners: If your partner is doing the perineal massage, follow the same basic instructions as previously noted. However, your partner should use his or her index fingers to do the massage (instead of thumbs). The same side-to-side, U-shaped, downward pressure method should be used. Good communication is important—be sure to tell your partner if you have too much pain or burning!

Birthing Positions

Do you ever wonder why mothers lie on their backs to give birth? Traditionally, women in various cultures squatted while giving birth.

Being in an upright position allowed gravity and positioning to make the delivery easier. It is told that King Louis XIV had his mistress lie on her back to give birth in order for him to better view the birth. It wasn't to facilitate the birth, it was only to make him more comfortable and facilitate his viewing (typical!). Giving birth while lying on your back is difficult for delivery—it's like pooping in a bedpan.

Pushing in an upright position is great for both mom and baby. Being upright allows gravity to assist in bringing the baby down and out. Also, when a woman is upright, there is less risk of compressing mom's aorta blood vessel. So there's a better oxygen supply to the baby. Upright positioning also helps the uterus contract more strongly and efficiently and helps the baby get in a better position to pass through the pelvis. X-rays have also shown that the actual dimensions of the pelvic outlet become wider in the squatting and kneeling/hands–knees positions. This is good news for both mom and baby.

Your physical therapist can help you find the best birthing position for you. By using sticker electrodes on your pelvic floor muscles, your muscle activity can be measured with computerized biofeedback. You can practice bearing down, like you are pushing out your baby. It can be determined whether your pelvic floor muscles are most relaxed in a squat position, lying on your side, standing, or lying on your back. The more relaxed they are, the less trauma there will be to the muscles.

Of course this won't matter if your medical team needs you to lie on your back throughout your labor. But if you have options, we can help you find the best birthing position.

Labor Positions

Even though there are great benefits to pushing in the upright position, most women in the United States give birth either lying on their backs (57%) or in a semi-sitting/lying position with the head of the bed raised up (35%). A small minority of women give birth in alternative positions such as side lying (4%), squatting or sitting (3%), or hands-knees position (1%).

Squatting

Squatting to give birth is an option in delivery rooms and birthing centers. Most delivery rooms have a "squat bar" that you can hold on to help you position yourself for a squatting birth. Here are some exercises that you can do in order to get your legs ready for this feat.

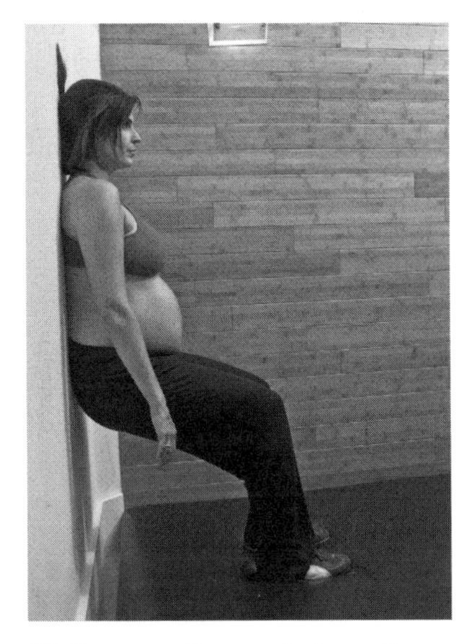

Wall squats for quad strengthening in preparation for delivery

Wall squat

- Lean against the wall and step your feet out in front of you.
- Slide down the wall (it doesn't have to be very far down) and hold the position for just a few seconds. Keep breathing!
- Really tighten your butt muscles and your thigh muscles to support you.
- Further tighten these muscles to push you back up to standing.
- Do 10 repetitions and see how you feel. If you feel strong, do another set of 10.

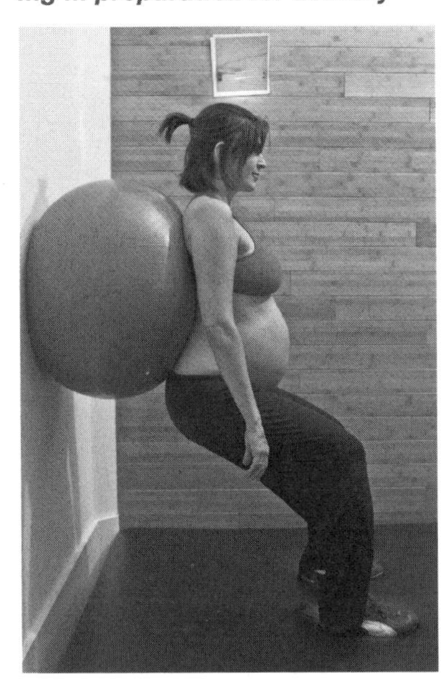

Wall Squats Using Ball

Wall squat with a ball

You've already practiced sliding up and down a wall to strengthen your thighs for your possible squat labor. You can now try using your exercise ball in this wall slide exercise.

- Place the ball between your back and the wall.
- Squat up and down. Make sure your knees don't move forward over your toes, as this will strain your knees. The ball helps to decrease friction behind you so you can slide up and down easier.
- Complete a set of 10 and see how you feel. If you feel good, then perform another set of 10.

Ball of Joy

Investing in an exercise ball or "birthing ball" is a practical idea. You can use it for many different purposes. It can be a seat for your sore bum, a surface for you to lean on, or an exercise tool. You can also use it to throw at your partner if he or she is not being sympathetic. Birthing balls are generally very inexpensive and can be purchased for $10 to $25 online or at a sporting goods store.

"Birthing Bar" or "Squat Bar"

This is not a place where you go during labor to drink excessively to numb the pain. A birthing bar is an attachment that can be added to most labor beds to help facilitate a squatting position. When using the bar, the foot of the bed can be dropped and the head of the bed can be raised. Between contractions, you can sit, supported by the head of the bed, and then during contractions move forward to squat, supported by the bar.

Sitting Upright

Raising the head of the bed and lowering the foot of the bed puts you in a more seated position. You'll appreciate letting gravity do some of the work here. And just like with the birthing bar, you can rest on the bed by leaning back in between contractions.

Birthing Stool

While this may not go over so well in the delivery room of your hospital (as most hospitals most likely won't have one), this is an option that you can use at your birthing center. If you want to push out poop, you sit on a toilet. Sitting on a birthing stool is kind of the same idea, except that you are pushing out a baby. The low height of the stool flexes your legs and expands the size of your pelvis. The upright position helps use gravity to promote the downward movement of the baby. As with the other positions, you can always lean back and rest in between contractions.

Kneeling

You can also attempt to push while in a kneeling position. You can use a birthing ball or the side of your bed to support your upper body. While you are pushing, bring your knees up and lower your butt slightly as you push. In between pushing, you can drape yourself over the bed or birthing ball to rest and relax. Here is another good use for your birthing ball.

Side Lying with Leg Lifted

Gravity is not at work here and you'll need someone to support your top leg while you are pushing. However, this position is helpful for a number of reasons. Lying on your left side helps blood flow since the baby is not pushing on the inferior vena cava blood vessel. If you have back pain, this position allows you to stay off your back while you are pushing. If you are experiencing pubic symphysis pain, being on your side pulls on your pelvic bones less, relieving strain on your pubic symphysis. We can't promise your doctor or midwife will be so fond of this position.

Relaxing the Pelvic Floor during Delivery

It seems like such a confusing contradiction: Push! Relax! Push from your abdomen! Relax your pelvic floor muscles! ... At the same time! ... And don't forget to breathe!

It's a lot to think about. As if you don't already have a lot going on at this moment.

How do you relax your pelvic floor muscles when everyone has been telling you to squeeze them during pregnancy so you don't leak? How do you relax them when a small human being is trying to pass through them? Let's practice:

This is a good time to use your exercise ball. Make sure you are using it near a wall or sturdy piece of furniture that you can hold on to in case you lose your balance.

- Sit on the ball.
- Put your weight through your pelvis on the ball, not your feet.
- Feel your "sit bones" melt into the ball. If you are sitting with good posture, they should be right under you. To make sure, put your hands under your butt and move the muscles out of the way. Shimmy side-to-side or forward and back until you feel these bones. Make sure your body weight is over them, and not in front or behind the bones.
- Feel the muscles in between your sit bones melt into the ball also.
- Imagine your pelvis is just like a flower that is opening up and blooming.
- Focus on your breathing. Take long, slow, deep breaths. With each exhale, imagine letting go of all the tension in your pelvis—as if your muscle fibers are limp spaghetti noodles.

When you are pushing, you want to make sure that you are still breathing deeply. Pushing doesn't mean, "Hold your breath and bear down until you turn red and your face explodes." You need to breathe!

When the doctor orders you to push, you want to maintain your breath while pushing down from your abdomen. Contract your abdomen, bear down, and relax the pelvic floor. You don't want to provide any resistance for the baby, so allow the pelvic floor to be soft.

Labor

Lill was in labor for 12 hours. She was anxious to meet her little man and was tired of waiting. She loved the rocking chair that was in her room. She rocked, rocked, rocked back and forth during her labor. She even dozed off between contractions when they were infrequent. She previously practiced her wall squats and made sure she got her thighs prepared for her squat birth. However, she rocked for so many hours during her labor that when she was ready to "push" her legs were too tired to support her in a squat! She ended up giving birth on her back. For her second child, she was again ready for a squat birth. Her husband reminded her not to fatigue her legs on the rocking chair. However, this time she opted for an epidural so it didn't matter. She was confined to bed and could not feel her legs so squatting was again out of the question. She had another delivery on her back. It didn't matter. Her babies were beautiful and healthy. She quickly forgot about her original birth plan.

We want your labor to be as smooth as possible, however it happens. Whether in the hospital, birthing center, home, or taxi cab, these techniques will help you.

During the First Stage of Labor

Is your first stage of labor going to last three minutes, three hours, or three days? Your baby is either going to be eager to make his or her appearance or be far too comfortable inside the warmth of your belly to come out. During the first stage of labor, your cervix is dilating and you will be experiencing contractions. Since you won't be running to the hospital after your first contraction (or maybe you will!), here are some positions and things you can do to help ease any discomfort you may be feeling while you are waiting for your contractions to become more consistent.

While you are waiting for your cervix to dilate to that magic number of 10 centimeters, you can use your birthing ball to get your pelvis ready for delivery.

Try sitting on the ball, keeping your knees and hips separated wider than hip width.

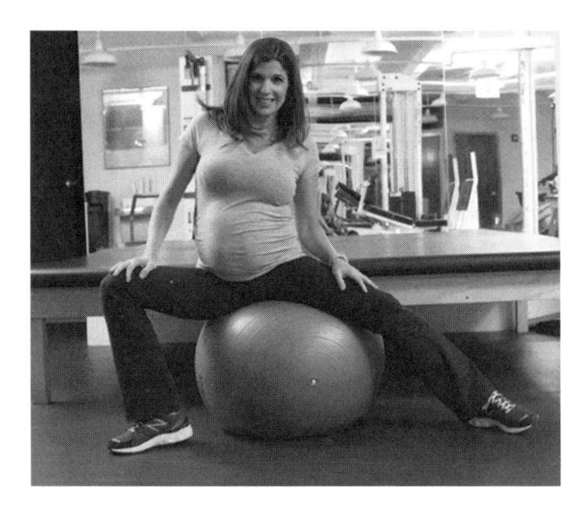
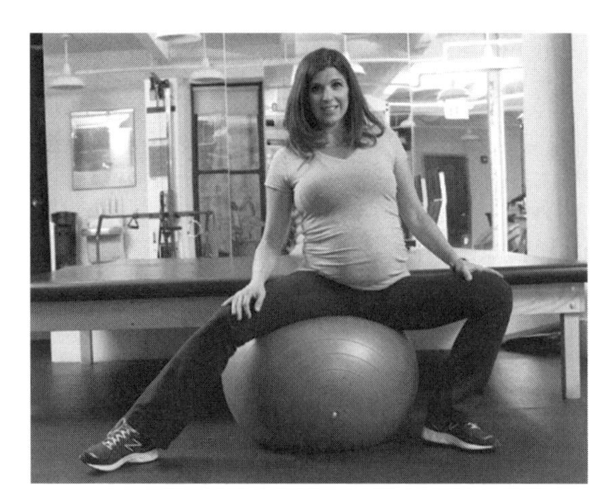

Using ball to massage perineum and open hip in preparation for delivery

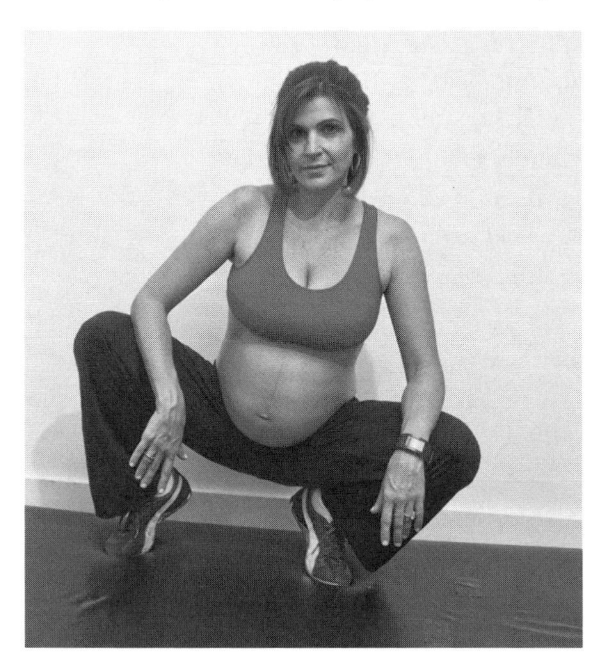
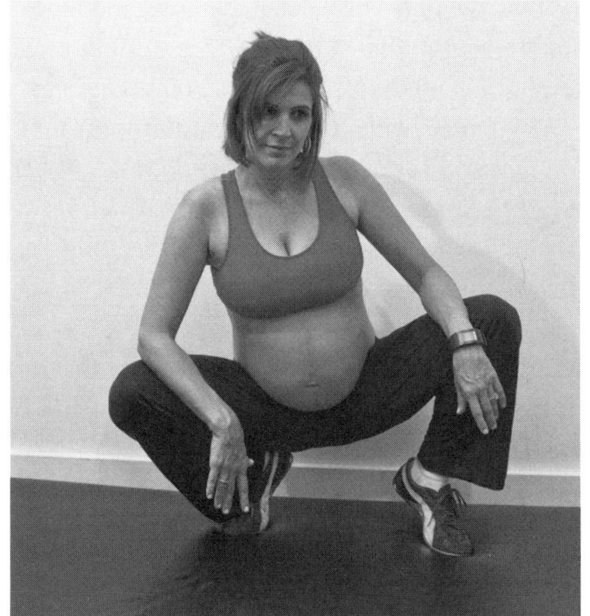

Rocking deep squat to open hips in preparation for delivery

Roll the ball under you, shifting your weight from one side to the other.

Use this motion to also massage the perineum and open up your hips and pelvis to get ready for the delivery.

You can also try opening your hips and pelvis by rocking side-to-side in a squat position. Deep squats may not be an ideal position for you because they increase the compressive forces in your knees. Please avoid this if you have knee pain. If you can, try this position for a short period of time to get ready for delivery.

Just as with the ball, squat down to the floor and shift your weight side-to-side.

Make sure to keep your knees separated in a "V" position and hold each position for a few seconds.

If you are having labor pains in your back, there are a few ways to relieve the pressure on your low spine.

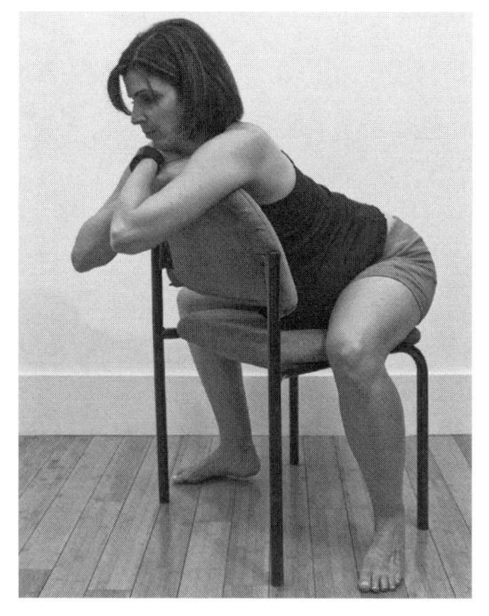

Straddling a chair to take pressure off low back during labor

Straddle a chair

Straddle a chair, facing the backrest.

Lean forward so that your arms/shoulders/torso are resting on the back of the chair.

Relax here for a few minutes and take some deep breaths.

Use your ball for support

You can also use your birthing ball to help unlock your lumbar spine.

Start on all fours with your ball in front of you.

Roll your ball under your torso and rest your arms/shoulders/upper body on the ball and lean into it.

Rest here for a few minutes and feel the relief on your low back.

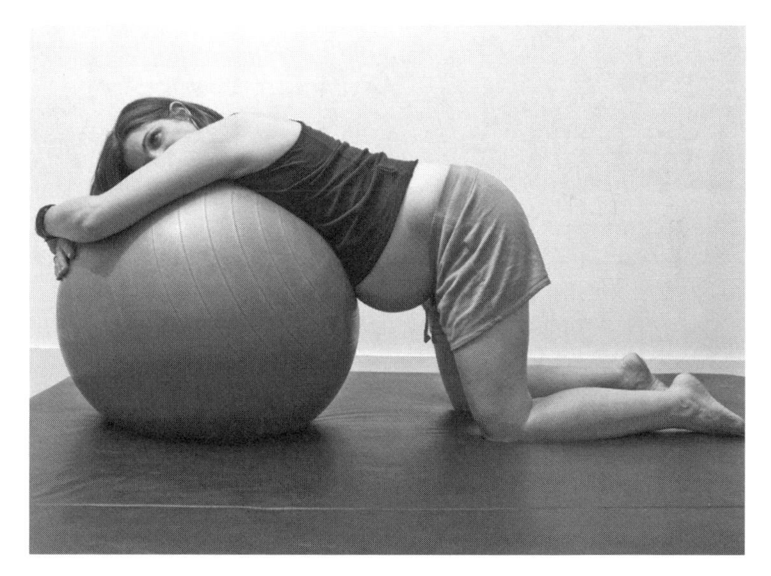

Using a ball to relieve back pain during labor

Use your partner

Feel free to use your partner for some support.

Face your partner and then wrap your arms around his or her neck/shoulders. Maybe because you want someone to hold you up. Maybe because you want someone to hug. And maybe because you want someone to strangle for the annoying coaching.

Tell your partner to step back or lean back to support you.

Lean your weight forward to relieve the pressure on your back.

You can also try the deep squat position (again, the *only* time we recommend a deep squat is to stretch the perineum to prepare for delivery) with your partner.

Sit in a deep squat with your knees separated and more than hip width apart.

Hold on to your partner and lock arms. Lean back to unweight your low back.

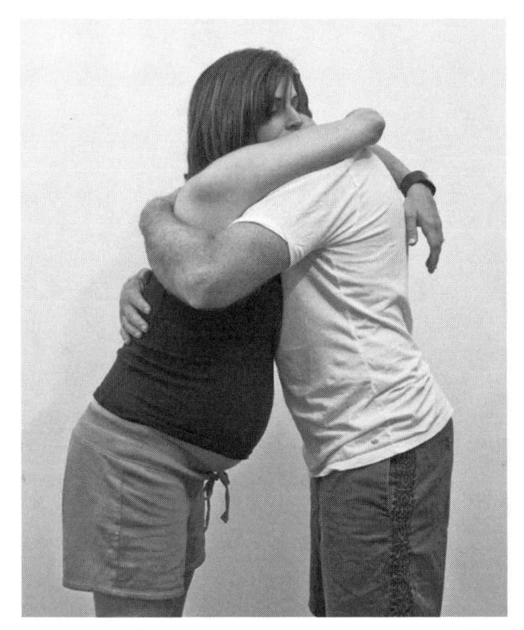

Using a partner to lean on during labor to relieve back pain

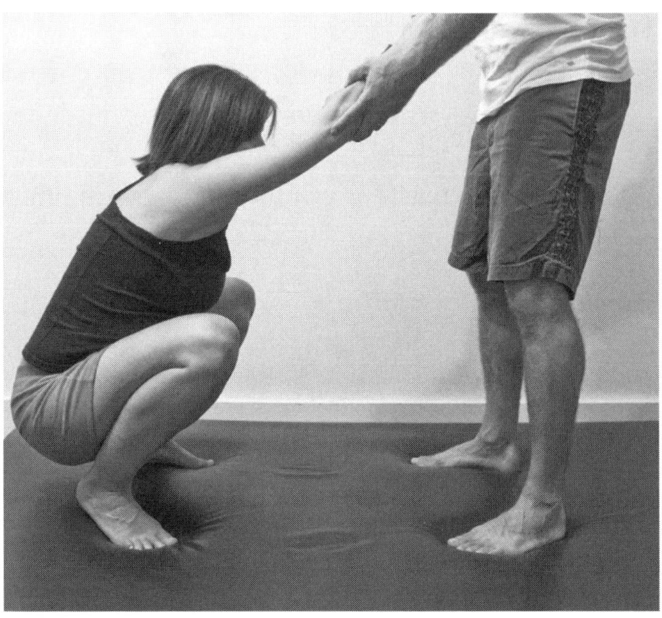

Using a partner to hold on to and lean back to relieve back pain during labor

You can also use your partner's manual skills to help relieve pressure on your back and pelvis.

Start on your hands and knees with your partner standing behind you. (Even though this is not an ideal position to be in throughout your pregnancy, it is OK to spend some time in this position during labor. The benefits of relieving the strain on your low back far outweigh the risks to the vulnerable abdominal connective tissue at this point.)

Your partner can then apply pressure on the sides of your pelvis and push inward. This compression relieves the stress on the ligaments in your low back and pelvis.

Many women tell us this is the most helpful trick during labor. It helps them through several uncomfortable hours.

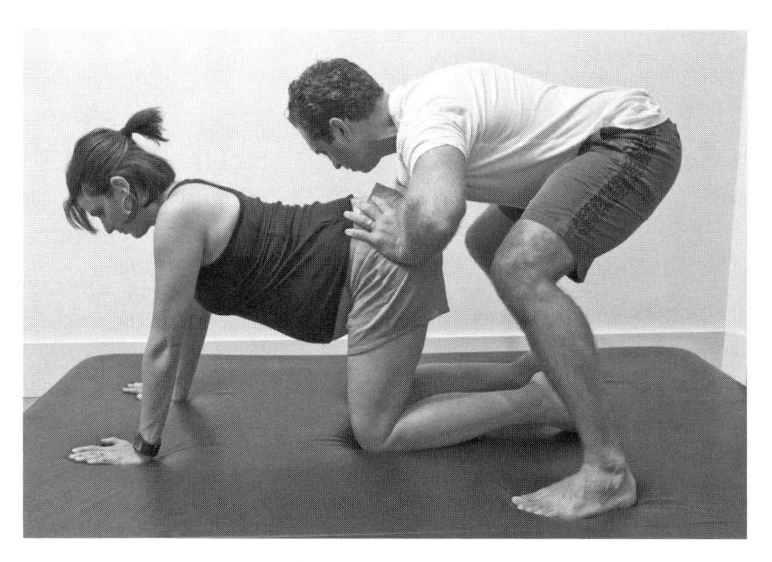

Partner applying gentle force through pelvis to relieve pressure during labor

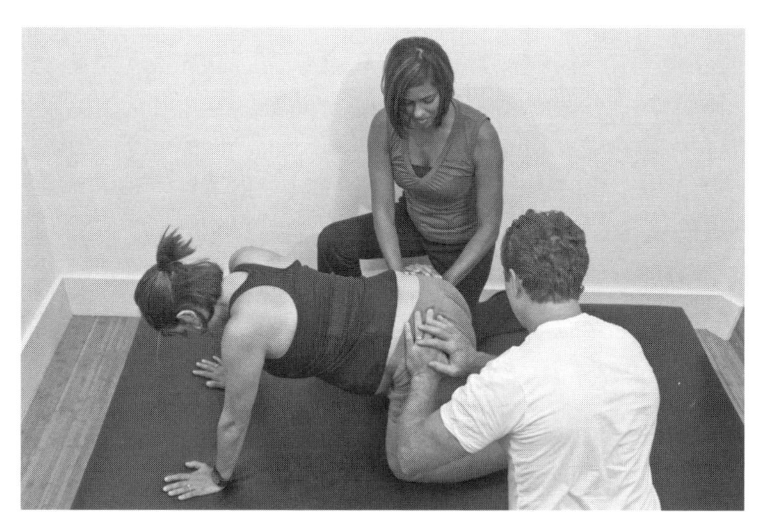

Two sets of hands applying gentle force through pelvis to relieve pressure during labor

You can also do this with the help of two assistants, if you are so lucky. Your doula, partner, family member, or friend can stand on either side of you and individually apply compression to each side of your pelvis.

Now that you're ready to meet your baby, you need to know how to take care of him or her. Read on to know the best positions and techniques for feeding, carrying, and snuggling up your baby. If you are having twins, we didn't forget about you. Read our special section for taking care of twins.

Walking Won't Speed Up Labor … Will Sex?

As much as we want to think that we have one up on Mother Nature, there's not much we can do to meet your little one faster. It is a myth that walking speeds up dilation of the cervix. Researchers reviewed the findings of studies that included thousands of women, and could find no evidence that walking reduced the duration of the first stage of labor. Dr. Laura Riley, medical director of Labor and Delivery in the Obstetrics Service at Massachusetts General Hospital, disputes this high hope of women willing to walk to the delivery room. Some women reason that gravity will lower the baby and put enough pressure on your cervix to prompt it to open. Dr. Riley writes that walking extra-long distances can start contractions by irritating the uterus, but it won't do much to bring on labor unless your cervix is already effaced. Plus, the contractions stop when you stop moving.

OK, so no walking … how about sex? The role that intercourse plays in the initiation of labor is unclear, but who cares? It may be due to the physical stimulation of the lower uterine segment, the release of oxytocin due to orgasm, or from the action of the prostaglandins on a ready cervix from your partner's semen. Of course, you should refrain from having intercourse once your water has broken, as that is a risk for infection.

CHAPTER 7

Safe and Helpful Ways to Take Care of Your Newborn(s)

Boppies, gliders, and ergos … oh my!

Let the fun begin!

So you are exhausted, sore, and overwhelmed to say the least. Remember all those experts on pregnancy that were trying to give you advice? They're back. Now you're being told how to feed, when you should or shouldn't go back to work, why your baby isn't sleeping, and everything else you're doing wrong. Well, don't worry. We don't judge. We just nag to make sure you are taking care of yourself. Please know, there isn't just one right way to care for your newborn(s). Do what is best for you and your little ones. Don't worry about what others think, say, or do. Just love your little ones and enjoy this new job, as challenging as it is.

Let's start with nagging you about your posture and body mechanics, once again. You're not alone. Take a look at the moms in your playgroups. Yes, newborns have playdates too. There are two common postures seen: Some moms continue to stand as if they're still pregnant. Their backs are excessively swayed, their pelvises tilt forward, their shoulders are rounded, and they lean forward when they walk. Others compensate for their postpartum abdominal weakness by leaning back. They rely on their spinal ligaments to hold them up. When you look at them from the side, their butts are tucked under and they lean their upper bodies back to make up for their weakened abdominal muscles. Neither of these postures is ideal.

Your abdominal muscles have been stretched out and worked out during the past few months. Remember these muscles play an important part in protecting your back and helping you stand straight. Stand

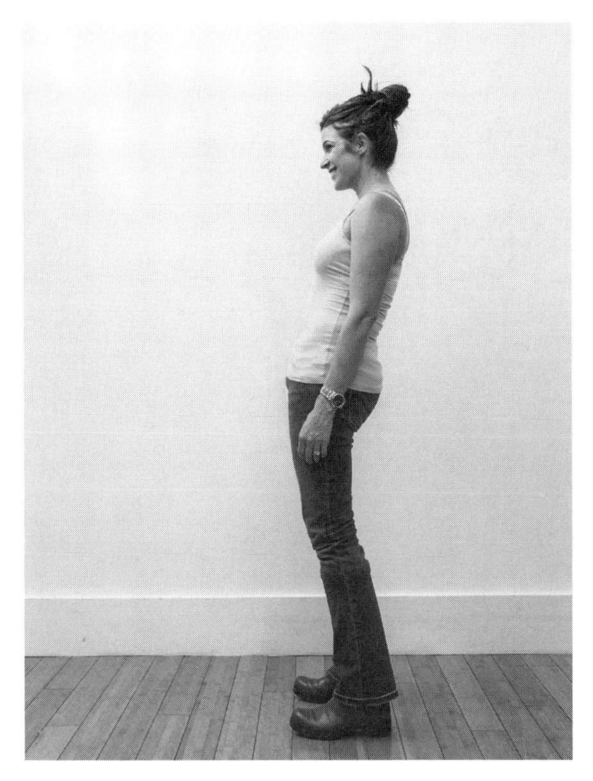

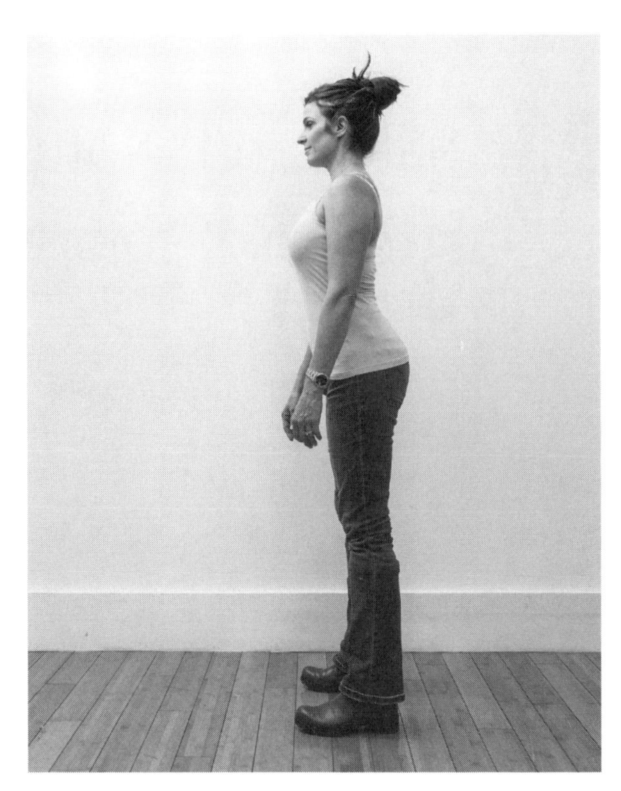

Poor postpartum posture

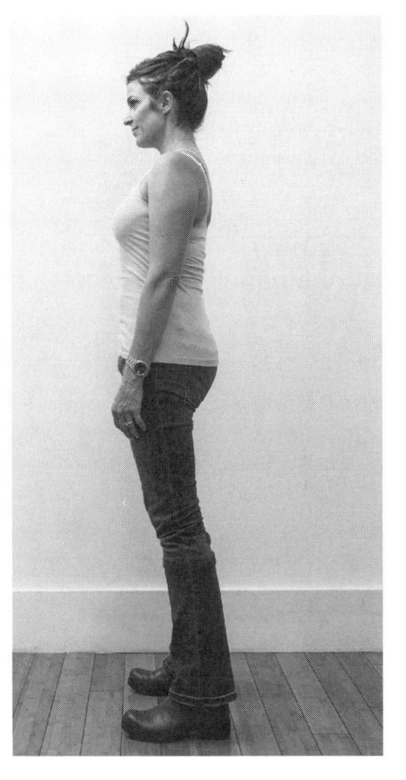

near a mirror and look at yourself from the side. Try standing so that your body is aligned in as much of a straight line as possible. Tighten your stomach muscles so that your hips are more centered and you are not leaning back. Bring your shoulders back. Try to keep your neck in line with your shoulders and your rib cage over your pelvis. Now here's the hard part—try to stay like that throughout the day.

Please remember, your pregnancy hormones help relax your joints so your baby can be born. It doesn't miraculously leave your system after delivery so your pelvis may feel loose and unstable for a while. You need to be careful. You don't have time for an injury.

Lifting

Whether it's a laundry basket, a box of diapers, or a child, remember to bring yourself close to whatever you are lifting.

Correct postpartum posture

- Stand with your feet wider than your hips to give yourself a wide base of support and good stability.
- Keep your back straight and put your weight through your heels.
- Tighten your butt, thigh, and abdominal muscles to power yourself up back to standing.

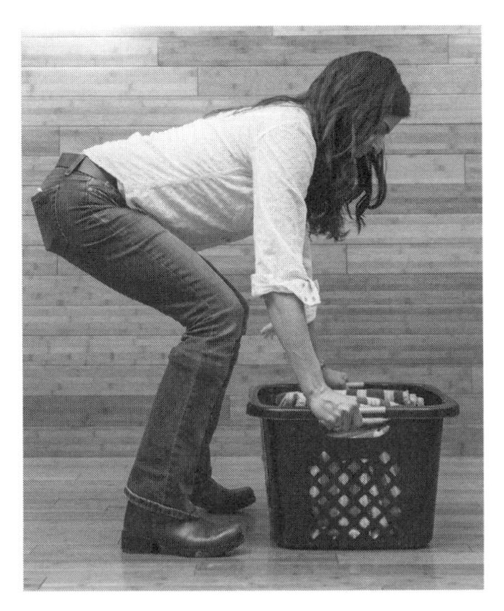
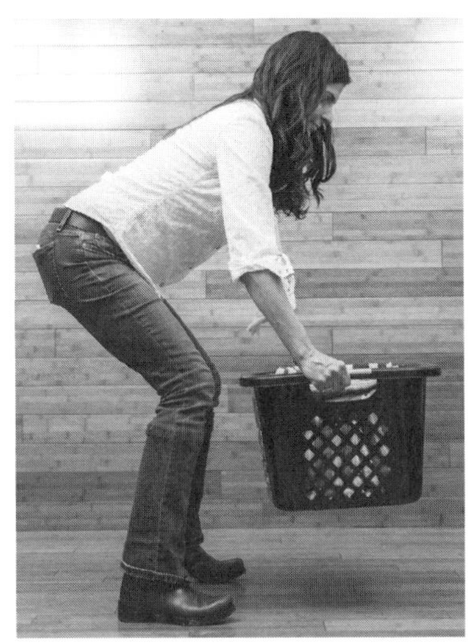
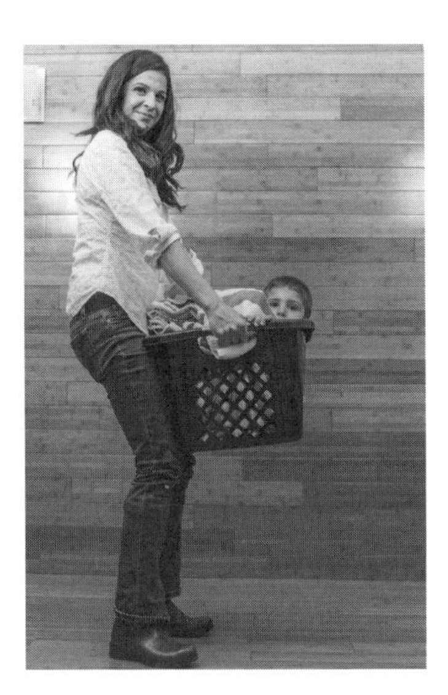

Lifting laundry basket: Good body mechanics are essential when the laundry basket seems a little heavier than normal

You may also want to try the"Tripod Lift"for picking up your baby from the floor:

- Place one foot beside the front of the object/baby and drop the other knee slowly to the ground.
- Lift the baby/object from the ground onto the knee, then into your arms while rising from the squat position to standing.

This won't be easy if you have bad knees, but it may be a nice two-step option for you if you can't squat to lift something.

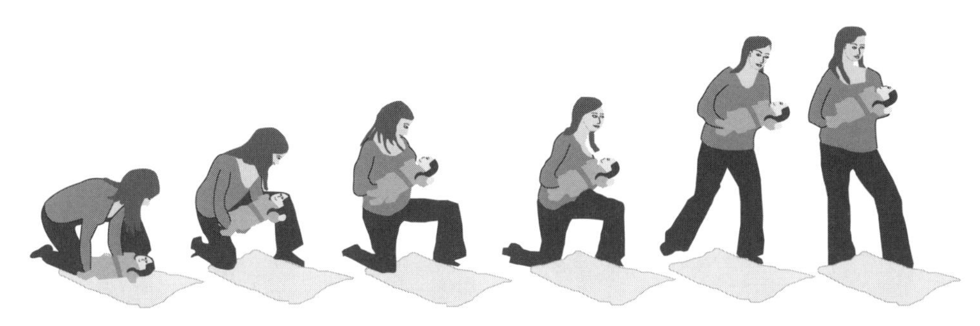

Tripod lift technique

If you feel as though you are straining your back to lift up, stop! Leave the object or child where it is and ask someone to help you. It's not worth hurting yourself and feeling sore for a week.

De Quervain's Tenosynovitis AKA Mommy's Thumb or New Mom's Syndrome

You may have one, two, three, or more babies or toddlers who you are lifting all day. Do you notice pain in your hand every time you make a fist, lift your children, grasp something, or turn your wrist? You may have De Quervain's tenosynovitis (dih-kwer-VAINS ten-oh-sine-oh-VIE-tis). This is a painful condition affecting the tendons in your thumb and wrist. It is often called mother's wrist or mommy thumb. De Quervain's tenosynovitis is diagnosed based on the typical appearance, location of pain, and tenderness of the affected wrist. To test yourself, try this:

- Fold your thumb across your palm toward your pinky finger.
- Close your four fingers over your thumb.
- Turn your hand toward your pinky finger (away from the painful thumb and wrist area).

This is referred to as the Finkelstein maneuver … no, not Frankenstein … Finkelstein.

If this hurts, you probably have De Quervain's tenosynovitis.

If you are experiencing this pain, here are some things you can do to relieve your symptoms:

- **Try to avoid lifting your baby with your thumbs and index fingers in an L position.** Many new moms lift babies out of cribs with their fingers around their backs and thumbs on their chests. This will put too much weight and strain on your thumbs. Instead, try to lift your baby by sliding one hand under the butt and the other hand and forearm under the upper back/head. Then bring the baby to your chest and use your forearms to support her or him. This will give your baby the support she or he needs without overtaxing your thumbs.
- **Try wearing a splint that immobilizes your thumb (called a spica splint).** This will reduce the inflammation and pain in your wrist and thumb. This can be worn while sleeping and during

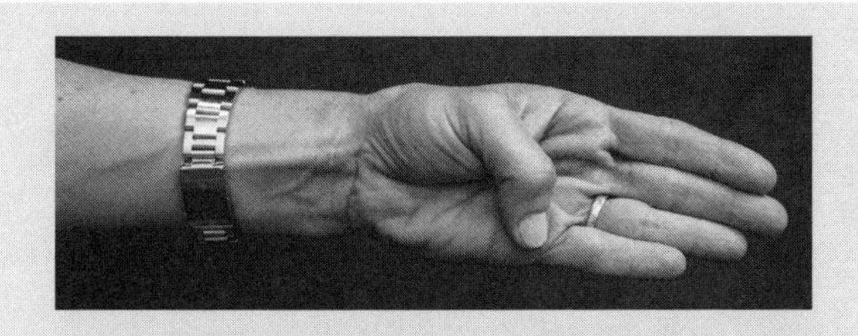

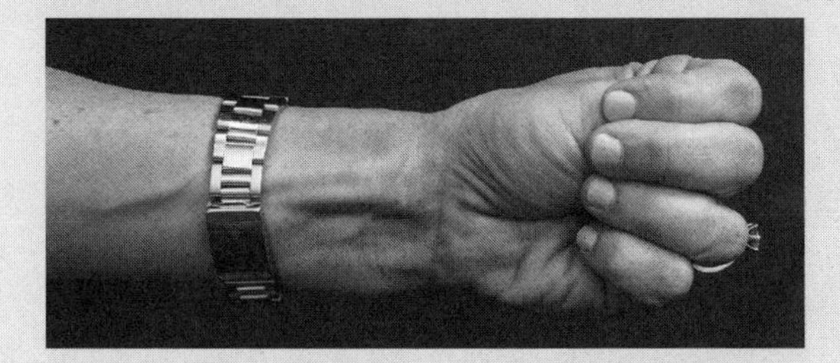

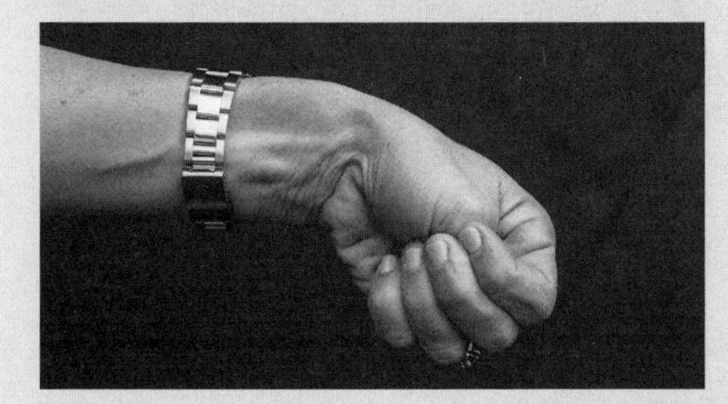

Finkelstein maneuver to test for De Quervain's tenosynovitis

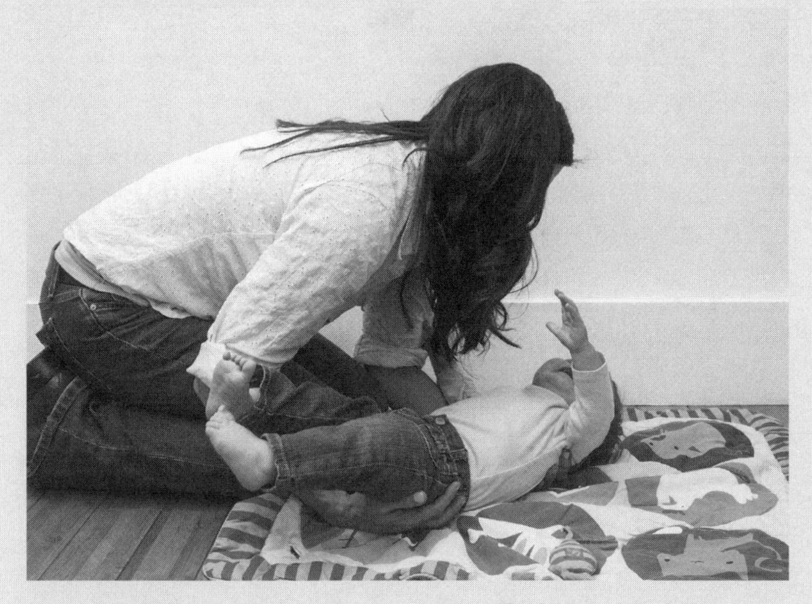

Alternate lifting technique for moms with DeQuervain's Syndrome (thumb pain)

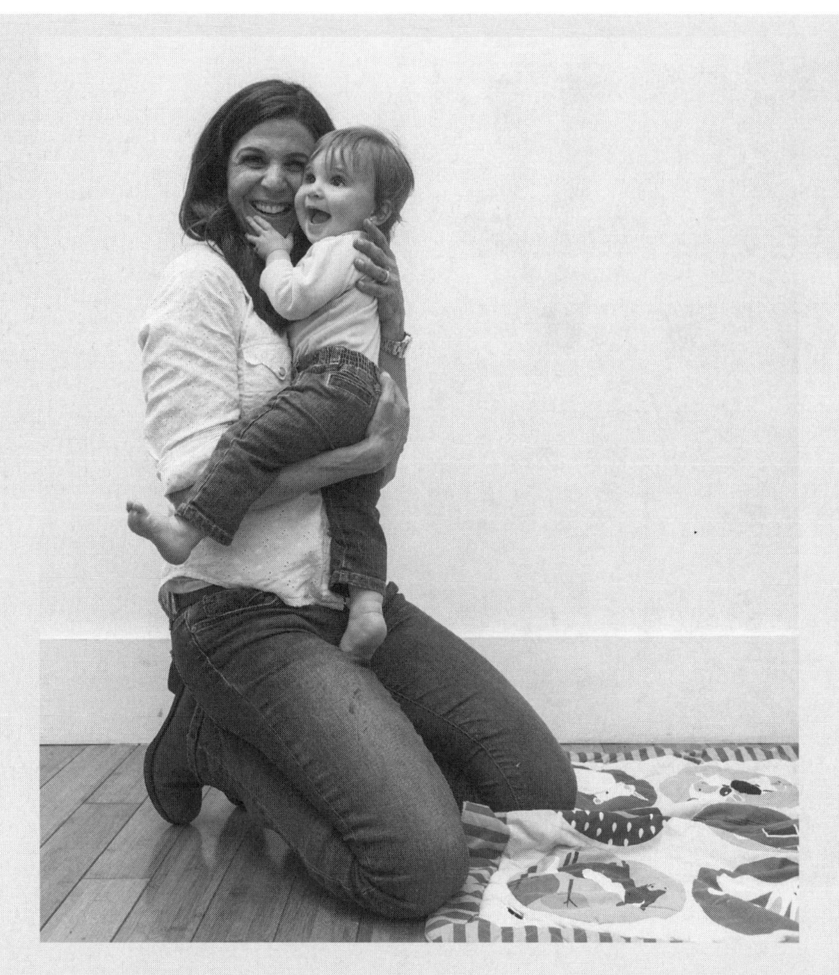

the day. Caring for your baby will initially feel awkward, but stick with it. You should see an improvement after several days of wearing it.

- **Rest.** Give your wrists time to heal. Besides changing your lifting mechanics, avoid excessive typing, chopping, smartphone swiping, and any other activities that provoke your pain.
- **Ice your wrist for 10 to 15 minutes throughout the day as needed.** Make sure you don't put the cold pack or frozen peas directly on your skin. Use a paper towel between your skin and cold pack to avoid an ice burn.

If these self-treatment remedies don't work, please contact your doctor and ask for a referral for physical therapy. We can help you, mama!

Breastfeeding or Bottle Feeding

There are several different feeding positions you can adapt to feed your newborn. Select what is most comfortable for you. Your two-week-old baby isn't too picky and doesn't have many requests yet. This is something you are going to be doing several times a day for several months. Make sure you are supported in a good chair with adequate pillows.

If you are nursing, bring your baby to your breast. You can use pillows to support your baby. If you are away from your home and don't have all your pillows and gadgets, try to sit upright or lean back slightly. Your newborn only weighs a few pounds, so it is manageable to bring him or her to your chest.

Don't lean forward to help your baby latch on. This will strain your shoulders and upper back. It's important that your baby is comfortable, but more important that you find comfortable positions as well. Most hospitals offer free lactation consulting services to help you with breastfeeding. It is difficult for many women so don't be surprised or discouraged if you struggle initially.

If you are bottle feeding, you also need to make sure you aren't straining your upper body to hold and support your baby. Use pillows, your knees, boppies, or the side of your couch to help you. If your baby is hungry, he or she will happily take a bottle in almost any position, so make yourself comfortable first.

Boppy pillows or any similar feeding support are very useful items to have. They are C-shaped cushions that wrap around your torso. You can prop up your baby on the pillow or let the pillow support your arms as you hold it. This will unweight your shoulders and release the tension in your arms. Whether breastfeeding or bottle feeding, try these positions to unweight your arms and shoulders:

Use a nursing pillow on your lap while sitting with your legs crossed or while sitting in a chair with your feet on the floor.

Lie on your side, supporting the baby with your arm and/or a pillow. This position will help to alleviate discomfort in your back or shoulders since you are not supporting the baby against gravity.

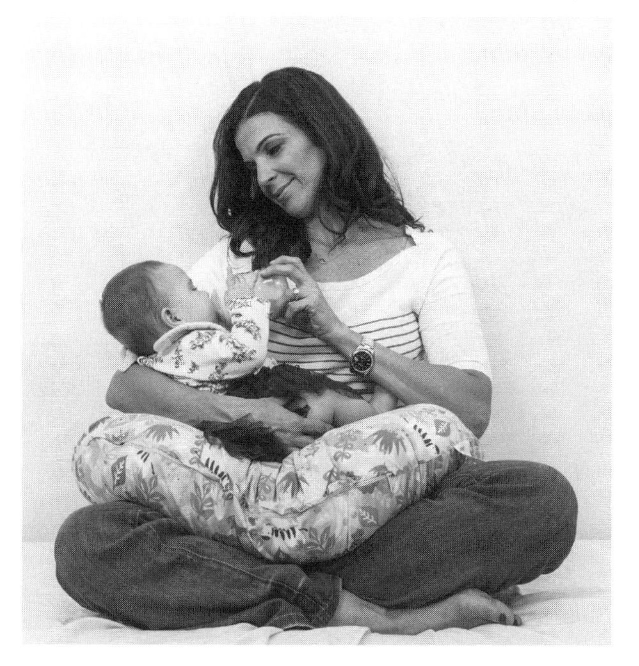

Feeding with a nursing pillow

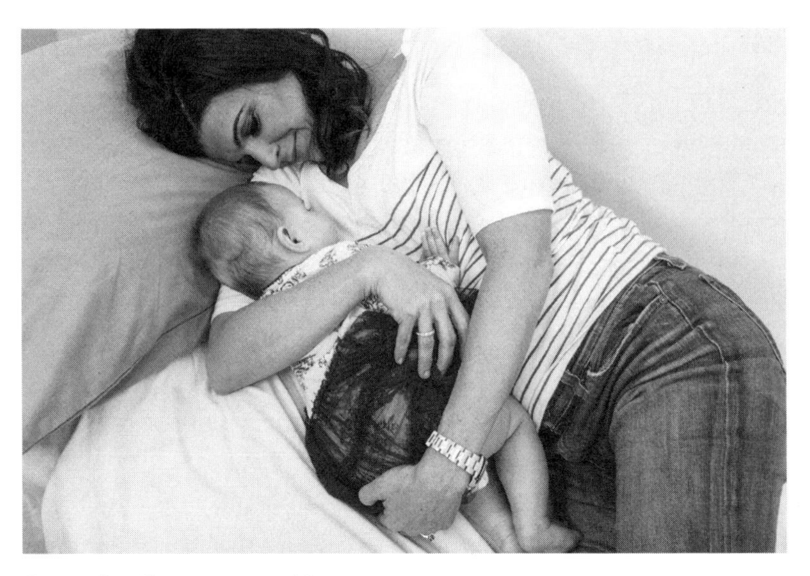

Breastfeeding on your side

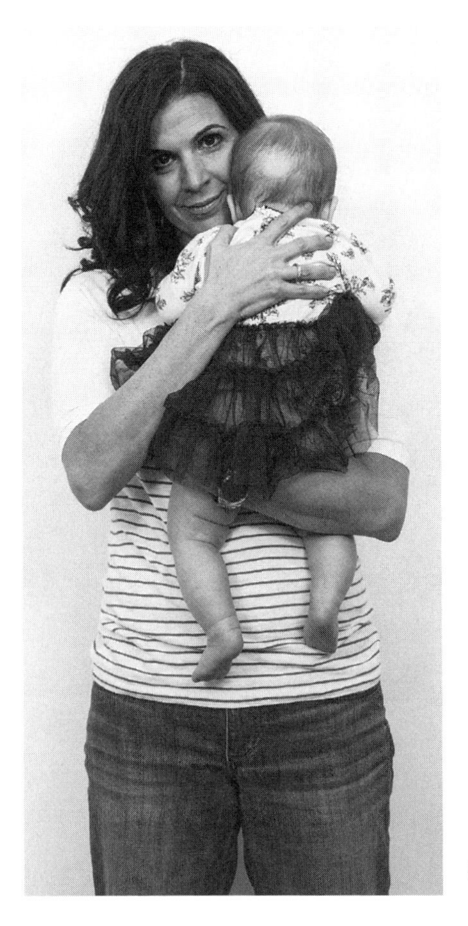

Carrying

Now you have to figure out how to carry this squirmy and slippery little person you just created. There are different options that you can choose from that are safe and comfortable for you and the baby.

Forward Facing or Rear Facing?

Just like a car seat, you may need to carry your little one rear facing in the beginning. His or her tiny neck muscles aren't strong enough to support the head, so you will need to support the baby's head with one hand as you carry with the other. As your baby gets stronger and no longer resembles a bobblehead doll, you won't need to support the head as much.

You can support the baby's neck and back with your hands, but make sure to not counter the baby's weight by leaning too far back. You aren't pregnant anymore so there is no need to stick out your stomach while holding your baby. Instead, tighten your

Carrying rear facing

stomach muscles to keep your center of gravity as central as possible without extending your spine (leaning back).

According to the American Optometric Association, babies' eyes do not focus on objects more than 8 to 10 inches from their faces (which is about the distance to your face when you're holding them) until they are three months old. So let them face you. They want to see you. They can't see much further anyway. Depth perception and color vision are present by five months so they may get more squirmy at this point if you don't turn them around. Their eyes want to explore their surroundings. You may no longer be the only person your baby has eyes for.

Forward facing

Once your baby can better support the weight of his or her head, you can carry him or her facing forward. You can support your baby by wrapping one arm around the chest and your other arm below, between his or her legs. Or you can wrap both arms around the baby's legs (which gives the baby ample opportunity to find, play with, and eat his or her feet!). Some babies are less fussy when you hold them on your side with one arm. Other babies will spit up as you're pressing on their digestion system, so be prepared!

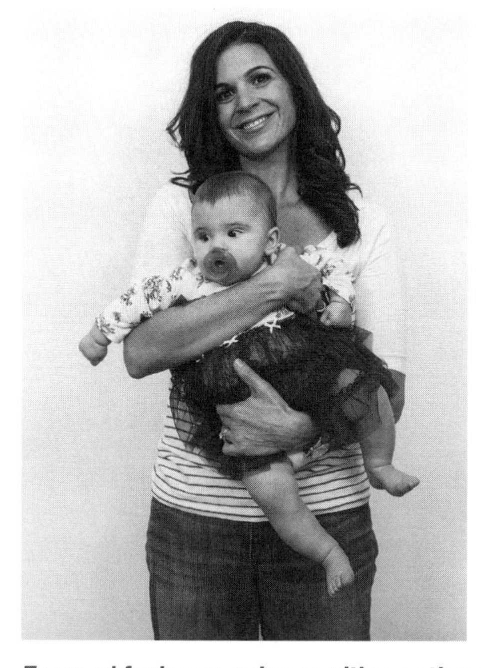

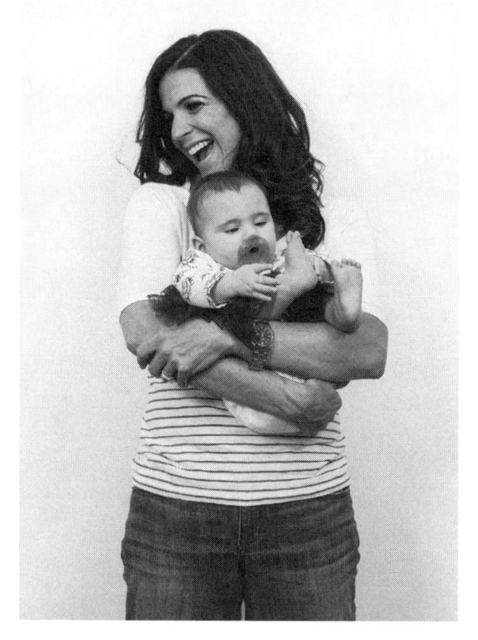

Forward facing carrying position options

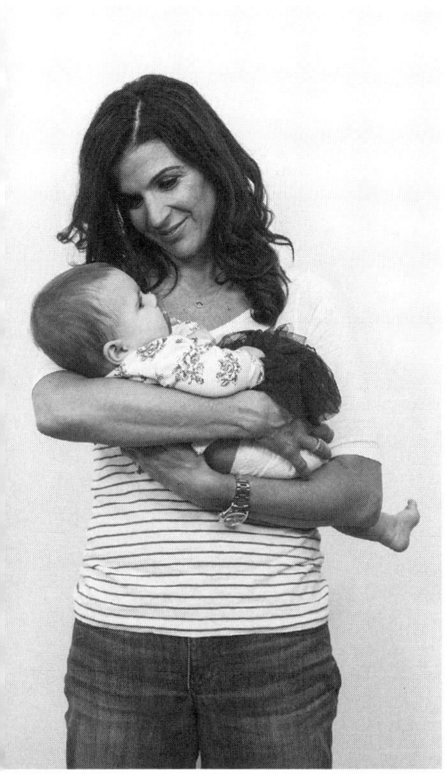

Classic cradle carrying position

On side

This popular hold allows you to hold your baby and also keep one hand free. The baby will be resting on your hip, but you have to be careful not to lean too much to the opposite side (see photos below for incorrect side-holding posture). Also, make it a habit to keep switching sides. Alternating sides helps you feel more balanced.

Classic cradle

You can opt for the classic baby cradling position. If you consistently use this position, remember to try and keep your shoulders relaxed. Don't hike up your shoulders because repetitively doing this may lead to shoulder or upper back pain. Try to support the baby with your arms and relax the shoulders.

You may have more than one child. The older one will be heavier, more squirmy, and probably more demanding. Weakness in your core will make you compensate and lean too much, which will put strain on your body. If you are holding your toddler on your left, you may lean more to the right. Or you may lean back too much if you are holding your child in the front. Tighten those tummy muscles in order to stay as centered as possible!

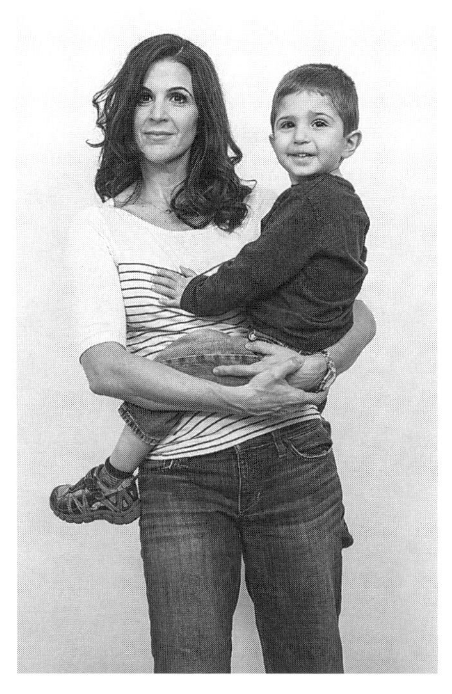

Poor posture (too much leaning to opposite)

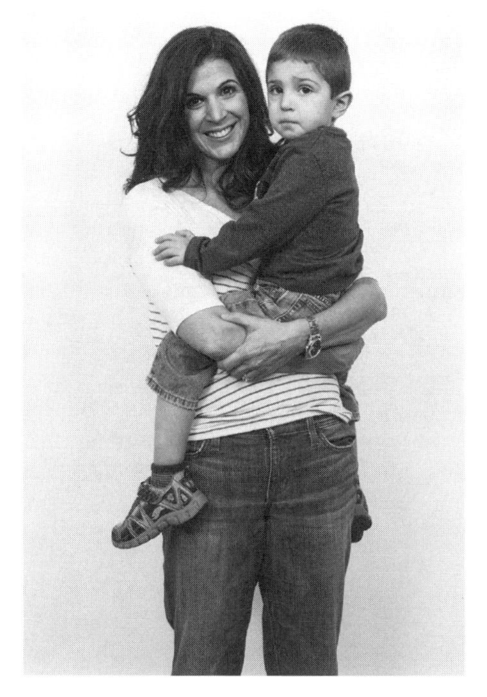

Correct posture (standing centered)

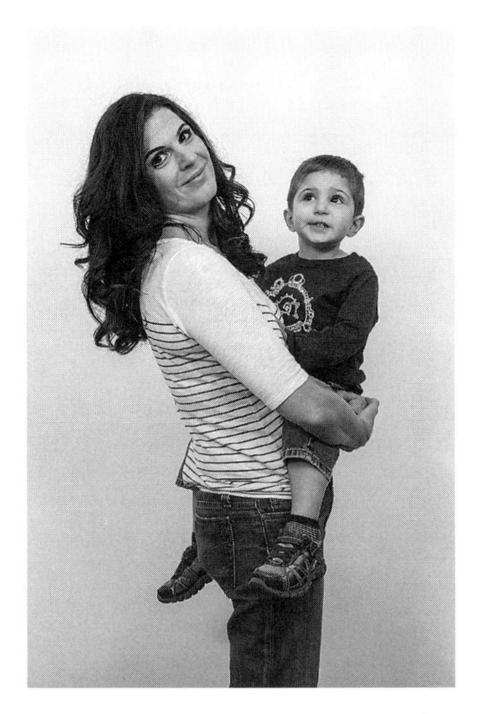

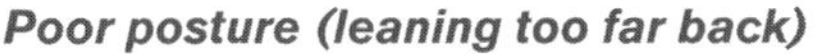

Poor posture (leaning too far back)

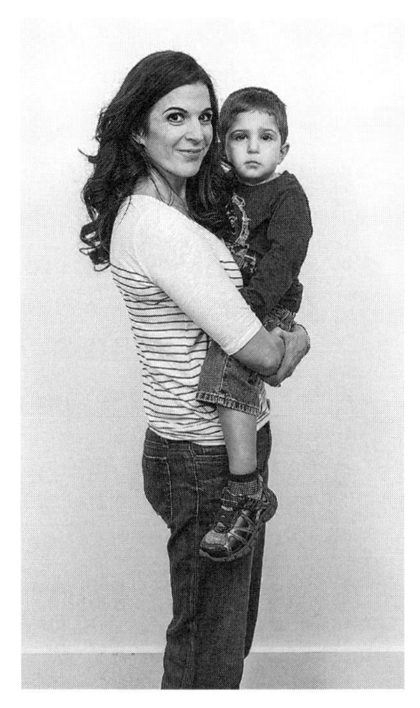

Correct posture (standing more centered)

You may need to hold both children at the same time. You know, when one is crying because ____ and the other is crying because of ______. You may just end up looking like the Help! picture.

If you are in this position, try lowering yourself to the ground so you are able to tend to both your kids and protect your back. If you tend to hold one child on one side, try switching it up. You may start to adapt to holding a heavier child on one side. You may get used to leaning to one side and may feel uneven. Try holding the heavier child on the opposite side to even yourself out.

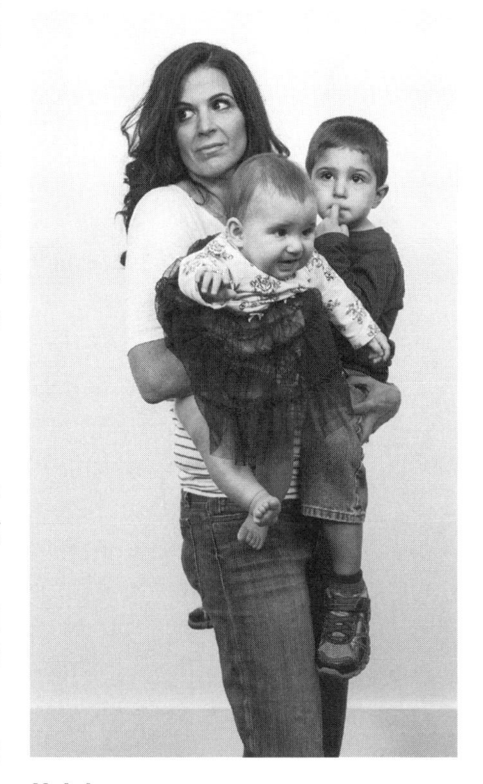

Help!

For Moms Taking Care of Twins

Working in New York City, we treat many patients with twins. As you can see, twins are on the rise. According to the Centers for Disease Control and Prevention:

- In 2009, 1 in every 30 babies born in the United States was a twin, compared with 1 in every 53 babies in 1980.
- The twin birth rate rose 76 percent from 1980 through 2009, from 18.9 to 33.3 per 1,000 births.

- If the rate of twin births had not changed since 1980, approximately 865,000 fewer twins would have been born in the United States over the last three decades.
- Twinning rates rose by at least 50 percent in the vast majority of states and the District of Columbia.
- Over the last three decades, twin birth rates rose by nearly 100 percent among women aged 35 to 39 and more than 200 percent among women aged 40 and over.
- The older age of women at childbirth in 2009 compared with three decades earlier accounts for only about one-third of the rise in twinning over the 30 years.

As you may guess, there is a lot of trial and error when caring for two or more. Whether you're holding them, feeding them, or playing with them, we will help you find the best system for you and your babies.

Feeding

Whether bottle feeding or breastfeeding, filling two hungry mouths can be challenging—especially when you're functioning on almost no sleep. Many new moms struggle with breastfeeding initially. Please don't get frustrated if this happens to you too. Lactation consultants can show you all the tricks. And if you are still struggling and you need an extra set of hands, just ask! Your partner, friend, or babysitter can easily snuggle up with a baby and help you.

Breastfeeding twins

Some of our moms nurse one baby at a time. Others have mastered feeding them simultaneously (called tandem feeding). And some moms nurse one baby while bottle feeding the other. For our moms that pump their remainder milk after nursing, feeding is time-consuming, so doubling up can be helpful. We remind our moms to change sides with each feeding. Besides the fact that one breast may produce more milk or one baby may suck more vigorously, you don't want your babies to have their heads in the same position with each feeding. Switching sides will help both their visual and cognitive development.

Using rolled up towels or pillows will give the babies the support they need. There are many pillows designed to support twins during feedings, such as Twin Z Pillow. This pillow has a middle leg that can be placed behind your back to offer support for your tired back. Wrap the two ends around and buckle them in front to secure the pillow around you. This buckle can be tightened or loosened, depending on the size of your babies. The sides have a firm slanted surface to position your babies comfortably at your breasts.

There are many ways to breastfeed two babies at the same time. What's most important is choosing a position that feels comfortable to you and your babies. Here are three popular techniques.

- **Double-clutch or double-football hold.** In this position, you'll hold each baby like a football at your side. Place a pillow on each side of your body and on your lap. Place each baby on a pillow between your arm and body. The babies' legs should point toward your back. Support their backs and heads with your forearms and hands, respectively. Their heads should be positioned at the level of your nipple. Alternatively, you can place both babies, head-to-head, on pillows directly in front of you. Be sure to keep their bodies turned toward you, rather than facing up. Use the palms of your hands to provide support for each baby's head.
- **Cradle-clutch combination.** In this position, you'll hold one baby in the cradle position. Your forearm will support the head and body. Your hand will support the butt. Your other baby will be in the clutch position, where your forearm supports the baby's body and your hand holds the head. If one of your babies has an easier time latching on to your breast or staying latched, place him or her in the cradle position.
- **Double-cradle hold.** To use the double-cradle position, you'll place both of your babies in the cradle position in front of you. Position your babies so that their legs overlap and make a letter X across your lap.

Whatever technique you use, make sure you're bringing the babies to your breasts and not leaning forward over your babies to feed them. This will strain your upper back. Grab more pillows if you need them.

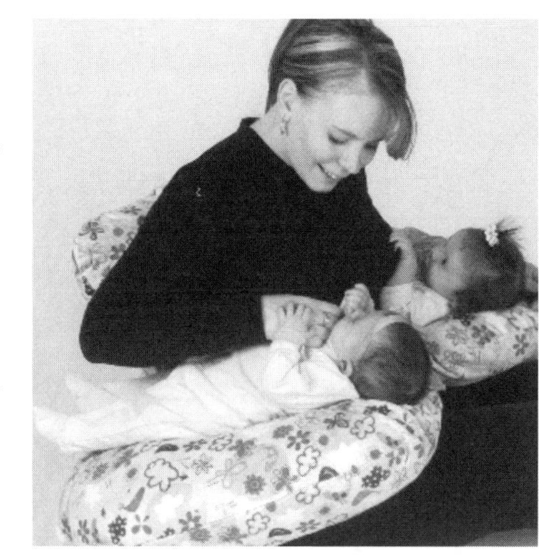

Twin breastfeeding position (double-football hold) using Twin Z Pillow

Bottle feeding twins

One trick for moms is to use infant carriers or bouncy seats. When the babies get older, you can use a floor seat such as the Bumbo or high chairs. You can also use rolled up receiving blankets to support your babies' heads or purchase infant head supports. Securing them in their seats will free up your hands

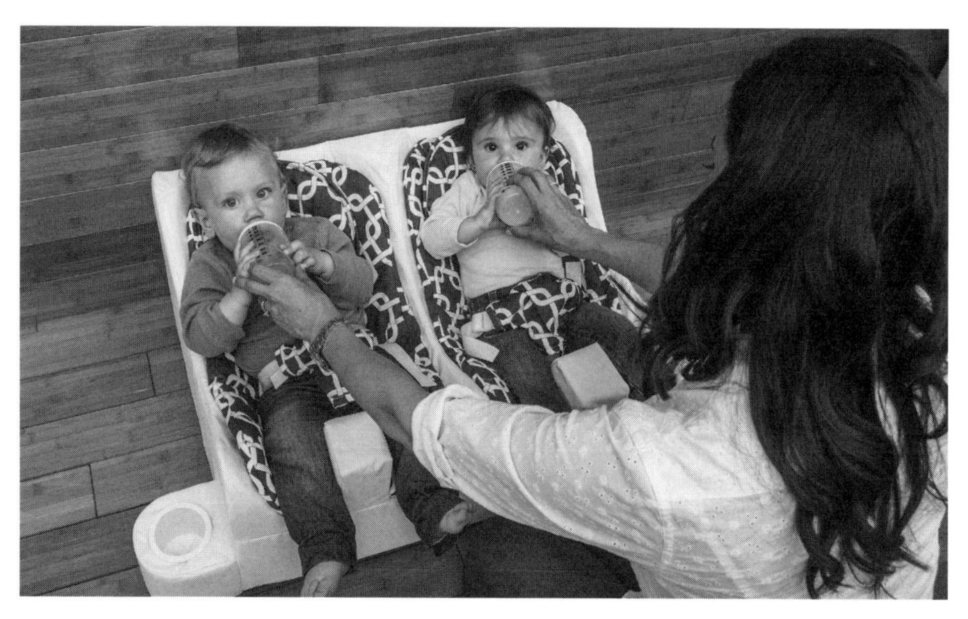

Table for Two for feeding twins

so you can feed them at the same time. We know many of our patients in New York City don't have cars, let alone infant carriers for cars. There are other devices that can act as extra sets of hands during feeding, such as the twin feeders from Table for Two.

Or you can use a twin nursing pillow such as the Twin Z Pillow.

Place the pillow on a flat surface. You can secure the twins on each side and sit in front of them, facing them to feed them. Or you can wrap the pillow around you with them at your sides.

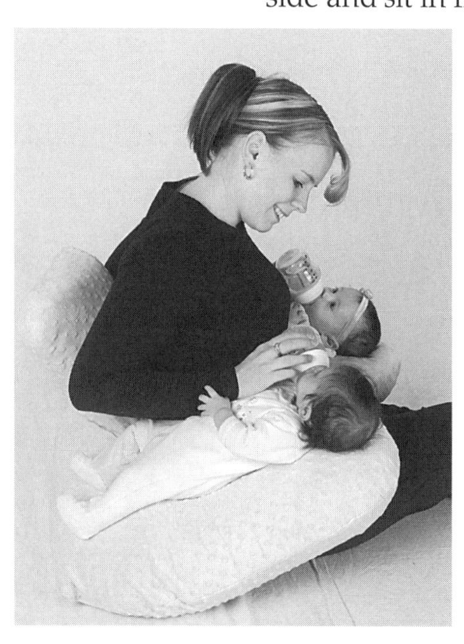

Twin Z Pillow for bottle feeding/positioning twins

If you don't have a device like this, you can use two individual nursing pillows. Make sure the babies' heads are supported.

Be prepared. Once you start, it becomes difficult to grab the bib or remote control you forgot. Set up your feeding area with some water, snacks, your phone, burp cloths, and anything else you need for additional multitasking. As if feeding two babies isn't enough to keep you busy.

If you are using infant carriers, nursing pillows, or bouncy seats, you can position them in different ways, whatever is most comfortable for you. Remember, most babies are too young to be picky yet, especially when they're hungry! So if you prefer sitting, then you can sit in front of them or between them (facing them) to feed them. Make sure you have ample back support.

You can sit against a couch or wall. Some women prefer standing and set up their babies on a sturdy table.

Once you get the babies set and secured, you can make the bottles. Begin feeding with your nondominant hand, so your more dexterous hand is available to help. Then you can feed your other baby.

Carrying Twins

Our postpartum moms have many different techniques for carrying their babies. While we can recommend different techniques, you need to do what is most comfortable for you. After all, you pick up your babies up to 50 times per day. Our patients often tell us about their back pain associated with picking up or putting down their twins.

Here are our tips to avoid back pain when picking up the babies:

- Engage your abdominals before lifting. This will protect your spine.
- Squat down to reach your babies. Don't bend down from your hips and arch your back. Bend at your knees and work your leg muscles. Lifting your babies 50 times a day will be a workout for your legs!
- Bring the babies close to you before lifting. Don't grab them while turning your body or with outstretched arms.
- Don't hold your breath.

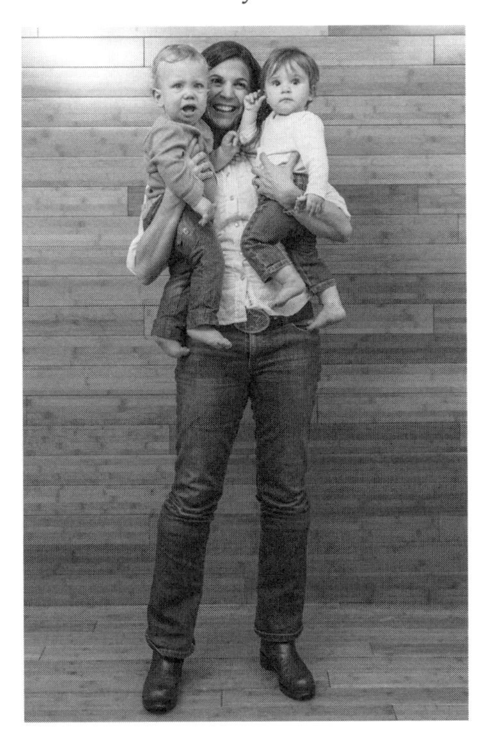

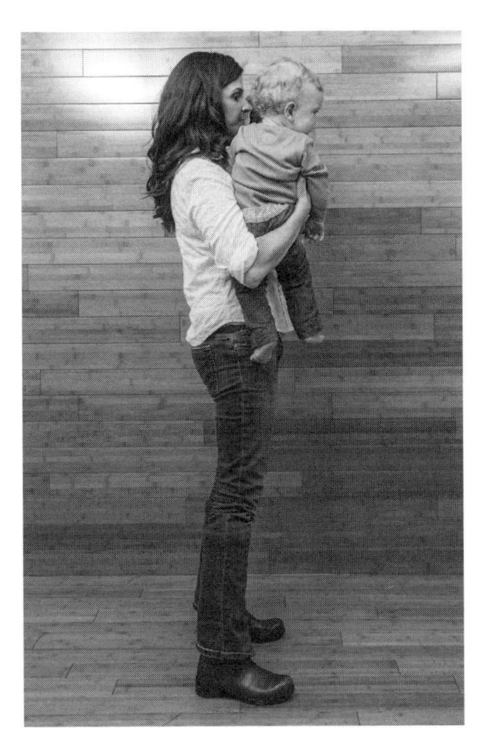

Carrying option for twins

Marie came to see us for an abdominal diastasis and low back pain after she had twin girls. She had two older daughters and not much help, so she got efficient at multitasking. "If I was taking the twins out of the crib I would move one at a time from the crib to my bed to dress or change them. I would hold both of them and move around the house. I was alone most of the time with them so if I had to hold them at the same time I got really good at scooping them up. I would pick one baby up with both of my hands and lean her on my one shoulder. I would hold her head and body with one hand and arm. To pick up the second baby, I would reach under her, cradle her head in my hand and her body on my arm. I would pull her up to my other shoulder. I also held them on my forearms in front of me. I cradled their heads in my hands while my arms supported their bodies. That was more tiring. And sometimes I even put both of them in a wrap to be hands free, which got to be way too heavy. I didn't drive much, but when I did I would carry two car seats, which were so heavy and bulky. I preferred the double stroller. I spent a lot of time that first year with them lying on each side of my huge twin nursing pillow. That was the easiest way to hold them both in the beginning. They would be at my side, in my arms, propped up by the pillow."

When Carrying the Infant Carrier(s)

If you're only holding one carrier, hold it in front of your body, using both hands to hold the ends. If you need to take two carriers, try to use a stroller. Carriers are heavy and awkward and even more cumbersome when you have a diaper bag falling off your shoulder. If you need to hold two carriers and a stroller isn't an option, make sure to pull your belly button toward your spine. Some of our patients wear an abdominal splint. This reminds them to engage their core muscles and helps protect their backs.

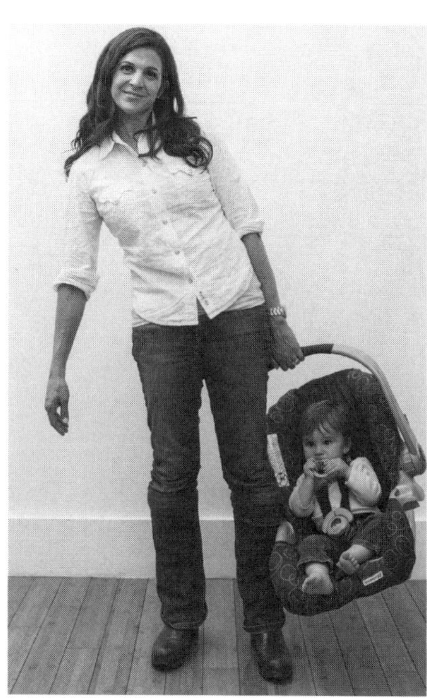

Incorrect way to carry car seat

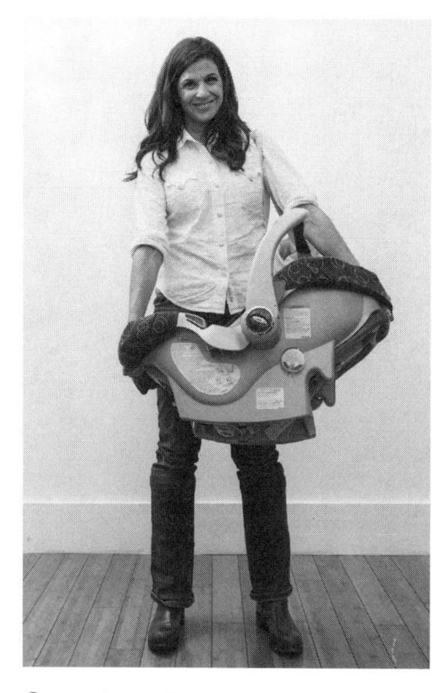

Correct way to carry car seat

If both hands aren't available to hold the infant carrier, try to keep your body upright and your abdominal muscles engaged as you hold it in one hand at your side. Don't lean away from it, as this could injure your back.

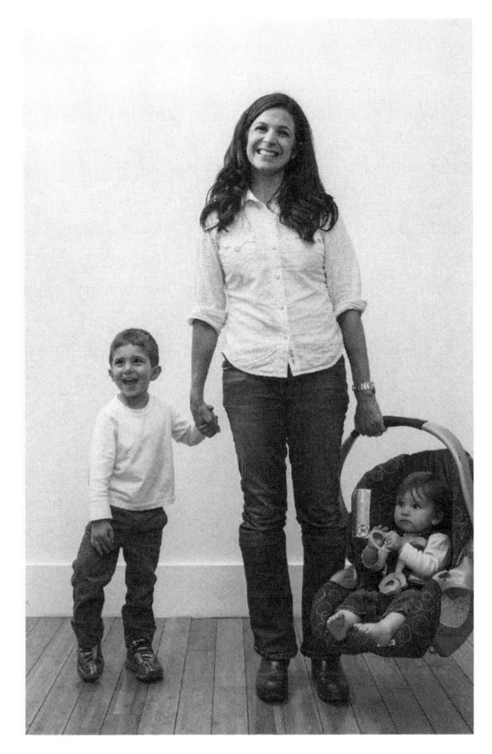

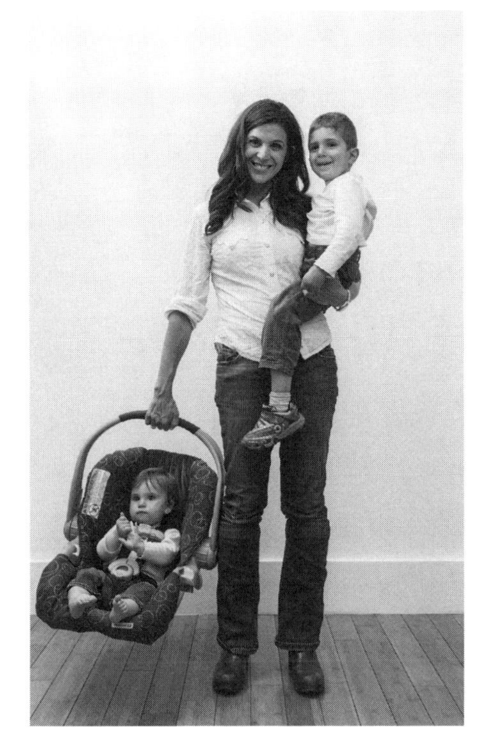

Correct ways to carry car seat in one hand and handling another child with the opposite hand

Slings and Carriers

Using slings and carriers to hold your baby(ies) is a great way to free up your hands while comfortably snuggling up your little ones. They are perfect for the multitasking mom and helpful when traveling, running errands, cooking, or attempting to pacify a screaming baby.

We advise our patients with diastases (abdominal separation) or pelvic floor weakness (those leaking urine involuntarily) to use a sling and hold their babies on alternating sides. Front carriers could make these conditions worse. This happens when the centered baby puts additional pressure on the abdominal connective tissue and bladder. Carriers and slings should not cause back or shoulder pain if used correctly and your baby doesn't exceed the weight limitation. Many companies offer YouTube videos to help you wear the carrier or sling correctly.

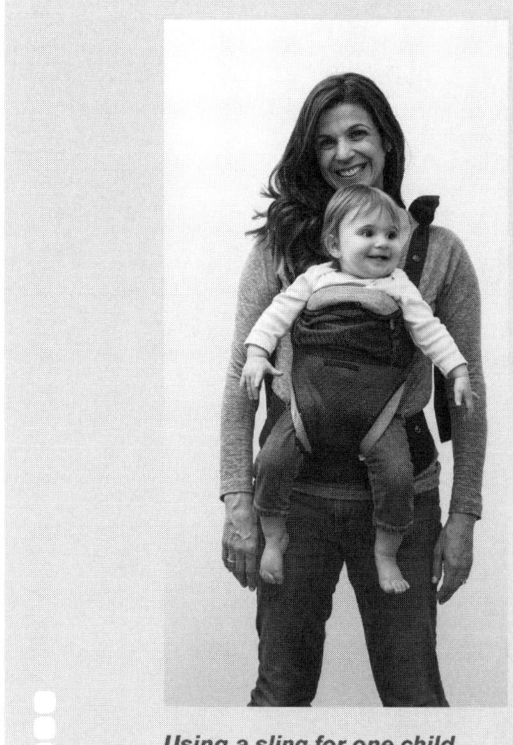

Using a sling for one child

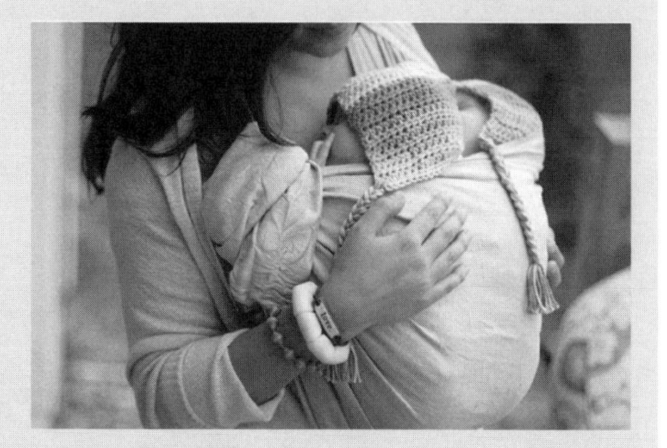

Using a sling for carrying twins (courtesy of Sakura Bloom)

We hope you now feel ready to take care of your newborn(s). You can't do this job well if you don't feel well yourself. The next chapter will help you regain your strength, fix your posture, treat your scars and your pelvic floor, and have you feeling like yourself again.

CHAPTER 8

Taking Care of the Postpartum Mama

How to feel like your old self again

Congratulations mama! You did it! And once again, some of you will have a postpartum glow. You have discovered love at first sight. You feel wonderful and couldn't be happier. Or, you may feel like you were just run over by a 16 wheeler. Life will never be the same. Well, you're right about that, but we can certainly help you feel better physically.

The Postpartum Check-Up

Your postpartum check-up occurs about six weeks after you deliver your baby. Your doctor or midwife may tell you to wait until this time before you start exercising or having sex. Your caregiver will thoroughly examine you, assess your well-being, and discuss your delivery. Please inquire about scar massage (for C-section or episiotomy). Once cleared, we will teach you how to facilitate the healing process. Please be aware of the following complications that can occur after birth. If you notice any of the following, please contact your doctor or midwife. Don't wait until your appointment.

Red Flags for Postpartum Women

- Heavy, bright red bleeding from the vagina that soaks through a new regular-absorbency pad in less than an hour and/or large clots (the size of a silver dollar or bigger).
- A temperature over 38° C (102° F) or chills/shivers that don't go away.
- Foul smelling discharge from the vagina.

- Pain during urination, difficulty urinating, or urinating too often.
- Breathing problems, such as shortness of breath.
- Lasting significant pain in the vaginal area.
- Flu-like symptoms and sore breasts, which could indicate mastitis or breast infection.
- Cough or chest pain, nausea, and vomiting.
- Cracked and/or bleeding nipples, which require the attention of a lactation consultant.
- A very red or swollen Cesarean incision, discharge or pus leaking from the incision, or continued pain in the incision.
- Pain or tenderness, redness, or a lump in the leg, which may indicate a blood clot.
- Sudden onset of severe headaches, blurred vision, or dizziness.
- Symptoms of the "baby blues" that continue after the second postpartum week and are getting worse. (Symptoms vary from feelings of inability to cope, frequent crying, mood swings, and fatigue.)

Stop Exercising If....

According to James Clapp III, an international authority on the effects of exercise during pregnancy, there are three absolute contraindications to *exercise* during the first six weeks after giving birth:

- Heavy bleeding (a pad every half hour)
- Pain (If it hurts anywhere, stop!)
- Breast infection or abscess

Relative contraindications:

- Cesarean birth or traumatic vaginal birth
- Breast discomfort
- Heavy urine leakage or pelvic pressure during exercise

James Clapp III states that the main goal of exercise in the initial six weeks after the birth is for the woman to obtain personal time and redevelop a sense of control over her life. To safely accomplish this, she should follow six guidelines.

1. Begin slowly and increase gradually.
2. Avoid excessive fatigue and dehydration.
3. Support and compress the abdomen and breasts.
4. If it hurts, stop and evaluate.
5. If it feels good, it probably is.
6. Bright red vaginal bleeding that is heavier than a normal menstrual period should not occur.

C-Section Scar Care

Scar massage

Women often worry about their C-section scars getting infected or how they can make them less noticeable. Some women don't want to touch or look at their scars and scar care is often neglected. But not for our patients! C-section scar care is important for several reasons.

- Scar massage will increase blood flow to the area, which will promote healing.
- Scar massage helps minimize the appearance of the scar and prevents it from getting bigger.
- Scar massage will decrease the pain, sensitivity, and numbness you may feel at your incision site.
- Scar massage will prevent the tissue from adhering to neighboring organs and connective tissue. (If you feel like your scar is stuck and the skin doesn't move well, you may have some adhesions.) Your uterus is *thisclose* to your bladder. In order to get to your uterus, your doctor or midwife will cut through many layers of abdominal tissue. These layers can adhere to each other in the healing process. If the tissues around your C-section scar are stuck together, this can affect the ability of your bladder to expand. So we nag you to drink lots of water if you're nursing and now you're running to the bathroom more than you did when you were pregnant. This happens because the scar tissue affects your bladder's ability to fill. That's a good enough reason to work out that scar.

Once your C-section scar has healed and your doctor or midwife gives you clearance to begin scar care, you will want to assess the tissue.

How is your scar moving? Is it moving at all? To check this, you don't have to even touch the actual scar. This is great news for those of you who are uncomfortable touching your scars.

Put your fingers on the area above, below, or on the sides of the scar.

Gently try to move your skin away from the scar in all directions. Try to move the skin above your scar toward your chest. Try to move the skin at the ends of your scar toward your hip bones. Try to pull the skin below your scar toward your underwear. Work your way down the length of the scar in this manner.

Don't use any lotion or oil and don't allow your fingers to slide over your skin as you assess the mobility of your scar.

Does the scar move easily? Does it seem restricted or bound down in some directions? Can you gently rotate it clockwise and counterclockwise?

If you feel resistance in one direction, that is what you need to address.

You can stretch your skin and underlying tissue into the restricted direction until you feel that the scar has loosened up.

Keep holding the skin until you feel a release.

Do this in any direction you feel resistance. In the beginning you should be working outside the scar. Eventually you will be able to tolerate working on the actual scar.

You should ideally be able to lift the scar and roll it in between your fingers. You want the skin at your incision site to move as freely as the skin on your upper abdomen, hand, or leg. Try picking up your skin (without pinching it) in these locations. Compare them to your incision site.

Skin rolling

Another technique you can try is skin rolling. Gently pick up the incision between your fingers and thumb and lightly roll it back and forth. The scar should be able to be rolled without resistance in each direction. Be kind to yourself. This shouldn't be painful! Only massage as much as is comfortable.

Does This Look Infected?

In the first few weeks after a C-section, it is important to monitor for any signs of infection: redness, oozing, swelling, or an increase in pain. If you notice any of these things, contact your doctor right away.

Episiotomy Scar Care

We gave you some tips in Chapter 6 on how you can try and prevent having an episiotomy. Maybe during delivery the doctor felt the need to cut you. There is a lot of information available on how to recover immediately from an episiotomy, but what about weeks later? Remember, the doctor had to cut through several layers of tissue. We don't want those layers of tissue to bind down and cause you pain.

Immediately after delivery, you can apply an ice pack to your perineum. The hospital gives out ice packs for you to use in your mesh underwear. Once you get home, you can make your own ice packs. Put some water on a maxipad, wrap it up, and freeze it. When you need it, peel off the sticker on the back, stick it in your underwear, cover it with a chemical-free tissue or small towel, and enjoy your homemade ice pack.

After obtaining clearance from your doctor or midwife, you can start massaging your episiotomy scar. Just like you tried to pick up and roll your C-section scar, you should be able to roll your episiotomy scar. You want it to be as mobile as possible. The more the tissue binds down, the more painful it will be to sit and have sex.

Using your thumb and index finger, try to roll the skin around your vagina back and forth between your fingers and pick up the skin.

It may be difficult since the area is small and not as easy to reach as your C-section scar. You can use a mirror or ask your partner for help. The goal is to break up any scar tissue and keep the tissue as loose as possible.

Pelvic Floor Strengthening

You need to begin pelvic floor strengthening before you leave the postpartum floor of the hospital. Your pelvis took a beating during your pregnancy and delivery. It is now sore, over-stretched, and weakened. If you had a vaginal delivery, it may also be healing from an episiotomy or tear. If you had a C-section, it is equally weak from supporting your growing abdomen for the past nine months. The good news is you do *not* have to wait until your postpartum check-up to start exercising your pelvic floor. You just have to wait until you are comfortable and feel physically ready.

Exercising your pelvic floor muscles will increase circulation and bring healing blood flow to the area. Sounds great, but strengthening these muscles after delivery is often difficult. The muscles are sore and weak. But you don't want to be one of those new moms that pees every time she jumps up because she hears her baby cry. Just because women often leak after delivery doesn't mean that it's *normal*. And it certainly doesn't have to last the rest of your life. So start squeezing!

You can start with the same progression outlined in Chapter 3.

Lying Down

While you are lying on your back, with your knees bent, practice squeezing your pelvic floor muscles as if you are trying to hold in urine. Hold for as long as you can.

Remember to keep breathing!

If you are only able to hold the contraction for two seconds, that is OK. Don't be hard on yourself. Remember you just pushed a baby out of there or underwent surgery. There is a reason you are weak. Your pelvic floor muscles are just like any other skeletal muscles in your body. The more you exercise them, the easier it gets, and the stronger they become.

As you get stronger, try to lengthen the time you hold the contraction. Increase the intensity of the contraction, as long as you feel you are contracting the muscles well. Pay attention to make sure you are truly strengthening your pelvic floor and not just squeezing your butt, abdominal, or thigh muscles. Try to keep those muscles quiet.

Once you can hold your contractions for 5 to 10 seconds, do some more. Attempt 10 to 20 contractions.

Sitting

Now try to squeeze the pelvic floor muscles while sitting. Being in a different position makes the muscles work a little differently. It's good to challenge the muscles in different positions, as we need them to work in different positions.

Once you can do this with ease, try contracting your pelvic floor as you march in your seat.

Hold one knee up for three seconds while squeezing your pelvic floor.

Repeat on your other side.

Try to march 10 times on each side.

Standing

Now try standing and squeezing your pelvic floor muscles. This is where it gets hard but you can do it. Once you feel strong enough, try these variations:

- Squeezing your pelvic floor muscles and marching. See how many times you can lift each leg before you feel yourself let go of the pelvic floor muscle contraction.
- Kicking your leg out to the side or behind you while holding your pelvic floor contraction.
- Squeezing your pelvic floor muscles as you stand up from your couch or while you are lifting a laundry basket. Always cue your muscles to kick in before changing positions or lifting something.

Many postpartum women leak urine when they laugh, cough, sneeze, or lift their babies. The more you exercise your pelvic floor muscles, the less you will have to think about recruiting them when you need them to be strong. We get it. There is nothing funny about peeing in your undies when you laugh.

Biofeedback

If you are having trouble locating your pelvic floor muscles, consider utilizing the services of a women's health physical therapist. We have specific equipment to help you find and exercise your pelvic floor muscles.

Your physical therapist may use a biofeedback unit with you. Refer to Chapter 3 for more information on biofeedback. Now that you have already given birth, it will be safe for you to use an internal vaginal sensor with the biofeedback unit.

Electrical Stimulation

Excuse me? You want to shock my vagina?

There is also the option of using electrical stimulation. Yes, this sounds very scary. I assure you that it's not. The biofeedback unit can not only pick up a muscle signal, but it can also deliver a signal. Delivering an electrical signal to the muscle can help you build awareness of these muscles. The signal will just feel like a gentle tingling and not like an Earth-shattering lightning bolt that will launch you off the treatment table. The electrical stimulation will wake up the receptors in the muscle and help strengthen those pathways between your brain and the muscle. Building this awareness will help you recruit the muscles and learn how to relax them as well.

Vaginal Weights

Another tool a physical therapist may use is a set of vaginal weights. I'm sure you never thought you would be lifting weights with your vagina, but these tools can help you recruit your muscles in a functional way. Using a vaginal weight while performing your pelvic floor muscle exercises cues your muscles to recruit while you are performing the activity.

The vaginal weight is about the length of a standard tampon, but slightly wider. There is a loop at the end of the weight that allows you to extract the weight easily. Sets usually come with a plastic cone and four to six additional weights to put inside it. This allows you to increase the weight you're using in small increments, ranging from 20 to 100 grams.

You insert the weight into your vagina and allow the loop to stick out. It should be inserted high enough so you feel your pelvic floor muscles supporting it but not too high, so your muscles just feel the loops at the end.

While you are performing your exercises, think about squeezing around the weight to try to keep it in. You can perform the exercises in all the different positions (lying on your back, sitting, or standing) and also while performing functional activities (lifting a laundry basket). Seeing a fluorescent colored weight fall out of your vagina while you are lifting a laundry basket is probably one of the more bizarre scenes you'll experience in your life, but don't be hard on yourself if it happens. It will just fall into your underwear and no one will know. Remember, practice makes perfect!

Work Those Abs

One of the primary concerns for postpartum women is getting their abdominals back to pre-baby form. Like pelvic floor strengthening, you don't have to wait until your six week postpartum check-up to address this. Performing abdominal exercises safely and with proper form is extremely important. We're not saying you should do 100 crunches the day after you give birth. It is OK, however, to start recruiting the transversus abdominis muscle shortly after delivery. Getting your abdominals back in shape may be a long journey, but you don't have to wait long to start on that journey. You want to reconnect with them right away.

You can do simple abdominal muscle-engaging exercises like deep diaphragmatic breathing (refer to page 78 in Chapter 1 for how to properly breathe from your diaphragm). Use your deep abdominal muscles to actively push the air out. Focus on bringing your belly button back toward your spine while exhaling forcefully. You can do these exercises regardless of the type of delivery you had.

Don't forget to engage your deep abdominal muscles as you lift your little one(s). Tighten your core as you get out of the car or up from the bed.

Here is a simple beginning abdominal exercise you can do postpartum while you are lying in bed:

- Lie on your back with your knees bent.
- Tighten your low abdominal muscles by trying to pull your belly button back toward your spine.
- While tightening your abdominal muscles, bring both legs up so that your hips are at a 90 degree angle.
- Keep breathing.
- Now put one hand behind your low back in order to maintain a small space there while you are performing this exercise. Make sure that you are contracting your muscles and not just rocking your pelvis back and forth.
- Keeping your abdominal muscles tight, alternate lowering one foot at a time toward the ground so that just your heels are tapping the floor. You can increase the challenge of this exercise by straightening your knee while you are lowering your leg to the floor.

If You Develop a Diastasis Recti

Refer back to Chapter 1 to learn what a diastasis recti is, how to tell if you have one, and how you can treat it. Studies show that 53 percent of women had a diastasis recti postpartum. If through your assessments you feel that you have developed a diastasis recti, please seek out the guidance of a health professional who specializes in diastases. You may also be experiencing back and pelvic pain since your abdominal muscles aren't performing their supportive jobs.

Many women splint the muscles back together to help the connective tissue between the muscles heal. If you had a C-section, you will want to wait six weeks and get clearance from your doctor or midwife. If you had a vaginal delivery, you can start right away. Please see the picture of a splint in Chapter 1.

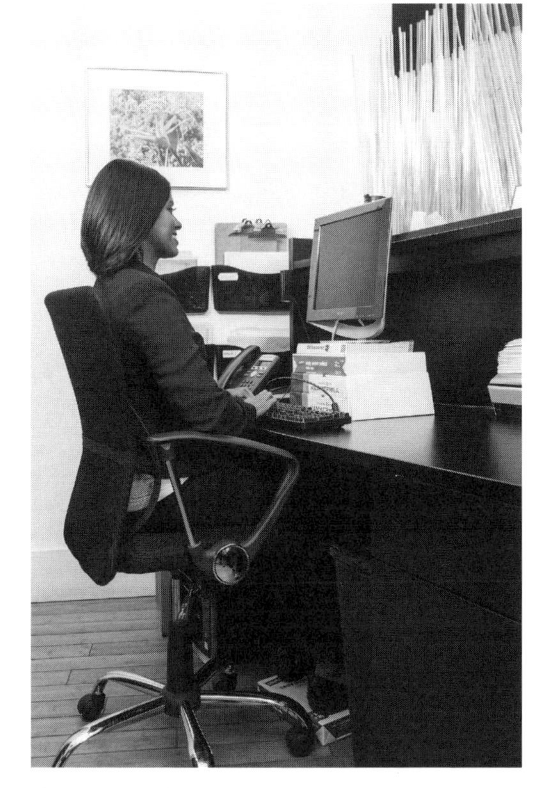

Proper monitor height at workstation

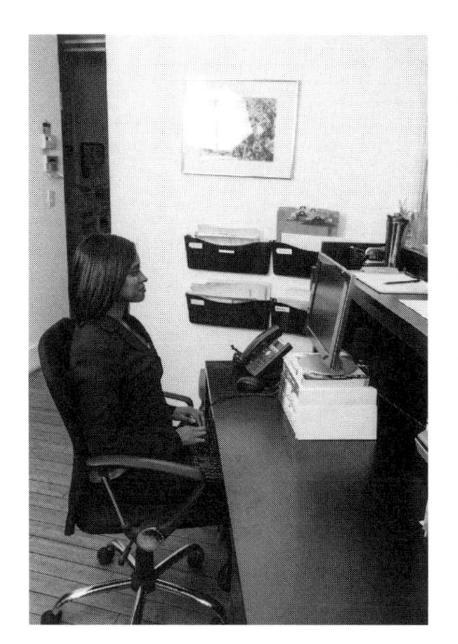

Proper workstation setup

Posture in the Office

Whether you are working part time, full time, or working from home, it is important to create a comfortable workstation. Habitual postures and repetitive movements can cause strain and injuries. Here are some tips for creating an ideal workstation.

We know you need to work with what you have, and that may mean a desk that can't be modified much or no desk at all. Here are some tips you can try. Do your best.

- Make sure your computer screen is at eye level.
- Try to create space at your desk or under your desk for your keyboard or keyboard tray. Keeping your keyboard to the side of your monitor will cause you to constantly turn your head at an angle and eventually strain your neck. So it is time to clean off your desk and place your keyboard directly in front of you. If your monitor is not adjustable, then stack some books or packs of paper under it until the words you are typing are at eye level.
- Make sure your arms are resting on the chair armrests. This allows your neck and shoulders to relax. If your chair is too big for you, you will need some support to take up the extra space. We frequently see this when we help our patients modify their workstations. Companies often use identical furniture for all employees—whether they are under five feet tall or over six feet tall. You will have to tailor your workstation to suit your size.
    - If you are too small for your desk and chair, you can support your feet with an adjustable footrest or books. You can use a lumbar support or pillow behind your back. This will help keep your body in better alignment so you don't overtax any of your muscles.
    - If your desk is too small, you may want to speak with your supervisor about switching to a new work setup that is better fitted to you.
    - If your chair doesn't have armrests, your desk is too tall, or you can't install a keyboard tray, you can type with the keyboard on your lap. With your hands on your lap, your arms are relaxed and you won't be holding tension in your upper body. Of course you can't do this if you still look at the keys when you type. This will strain your neck.

Your Home "Office"

You're lucky to have a boss that allows you to have a flexible schedule and work from home. You're not so lucky that your desk is also the kitchen table, platform for play dough creations, and prime spot for everyone to throw their belongings. This may not be the most ergonomically perfect desk, but we'll help you make it work.

- Purchase an additional keyboard for your laptop. You want your eyes to be level with the top of your screen and your hands to be relaxed. Since you won't have a keyboard tray, you can put your laptop monitor on a stand (or thick cookbook you never use) and the keyboard on the table or your lap. You should never have to strain your neck to read your screen.

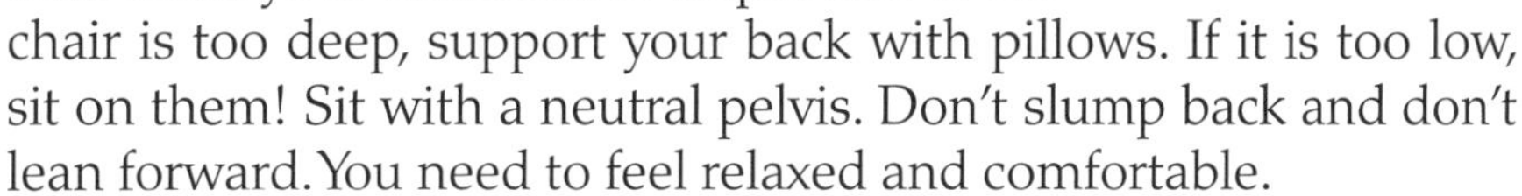

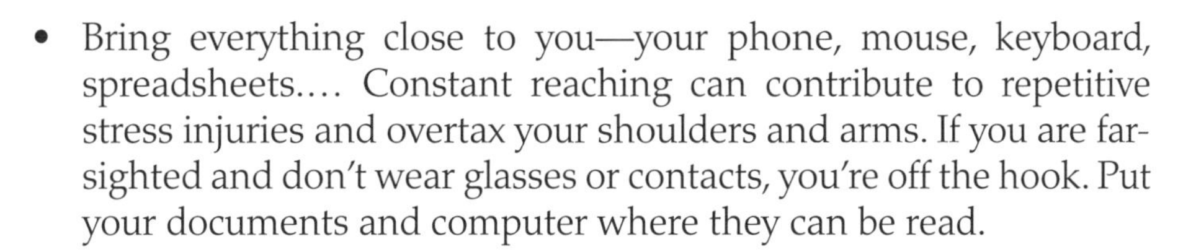

Home office setup

- You need to find a chair so your hips are slightly above your knees and your feet are flat on the floor. If you don't have a proper desk chair, you may need to grab some pillows from your bedroom to improvise. If the chair is too deep, support your back with pillows. If it is too low, sit on them! Sit with a neutral pelvis. Don't slump back and don't lean forward. You need to feel relaxed and comfortable.

- Bring everything close to you—your phone, mouse, keyboard, spreadsheets.... Constant reaching can contribute to repetitive stress injuries and overtax your shoulders and arms. If you are far-sighted and don't wear glasses or contacts, you're off the hook. Put your documents and computer where they can be read.

- Purchase a wireless head set to free up your hands while using your telephone. This will help prevent unnecessary neck strain from trying to hold your phone between your ear and shoulder. You need to be comfortable so you can focus on your work and not your sore neck.

Sex? Now? Didn't You See What I Just Pushed *Out* of There??

Your doc should give you the OK to resume intercourse during your postpartum check-up. Out of the 4 million women who give birth every year, half of those women experience some kind of discomfort when returning to intercourse after childbirth. That's a big number! A substantial number of these women continue to report pain even after one year.

Pain with intercourse is called "dyspareunia." This pain can result from trauma to your pelvis during delivery. You can develop scar tissue, adhesions, or tightness of the vaginal tissue. You can even have reflexive spasming of the pelvic floor muscles that may feel like a dull ache in your abdomen during deep penetration. Your vagina and surrounding areas may also be sensitive and inflamed after delivery. There are different ways to treat all of these conditions. The best course of action would be to consult with your physician and women's health physical therapist for appropriate treatment.

The important thing to know is that these conditions are treatable, but they have to be addressed very specifically. You don't have to suffer with painful intercourse forever. There is help out there for you. Don't be embarrassed to talk about it and ask for help.

Sex Toys ... or Therapeutic Medical Devices?

The best thing about going to physical therapy for sexual pain is that you acquire lots of naughty looking tools that you can now categorize as *"therapeutic medical devices."* You will need to hide these from your children of course, but not from your partner! Using these devices can be an enjoyable project for you both to work on in order to resume pain-free intercourse. Your physical therapist will give you the proper instructions, tools, and homework to treat your condition. You may consider speaking with a sex therapist to learn how you can still be intimate while working on your goal of pain-free sex.

Dr. Streicher, a leading women's sexual health expert, states that by the end of the first three months, 85 percent of postpartum women said they'd started having intercourse again. However, Streicher said data suggests that many women don't totally enjoy it right away. Thus, the "you're good to go after six weeks" advice that most doctors give to couples after a vaginal birth or C-section simply isn't realistic—or all that helpful, she said.

Dr. Streicher believes that the number one thing women don't expect is vaginal dryness. She adds that it may cause pain during sexual activity. The dryness results from a lack of estrogen, particularly among women who breastfeed. A good lubricant can help, but if the dryness persists, Streicher suggests talking to your health care provider about your options.

Intercourse is generally safe after any incisions have fully healed and you feel the delicate tissues of your vagina have healed. This healing usually takes several weeks. Equally important is feeling emotionally ready, physically comfortable, and relaxed.

According to a 2013 study, researchers found no notable link between a woman's childbirth history and low sexual desire, less than monthly sexual desire, and overall sexual dissatisfaction later in life. In the study, self-administered questionnaires examined sexual desire, activity, satisfaction, and problems in a multiethnic cohort of women aged 40 years and older with at least one past childbirth event.

"These findings provide reassuring evidence for women, who have had or are planning to have children, that neither the total number of deliveries nor type of delivery is likely to have a substantial long-term detrimental effect on their sexual function," the study's senior author Alison Huang said.

Are You Feeling "Touched Out"?

Stephanie Buehler, a psychologist and sex therapist, states that "Cuddling, breastfeeding, rocking and even changing the baby take a lot of hands-on care." Buehler advises that taking a break for a solo cup of tea or bath can help make whichever partner is feeling kind of "meh" about contact feel more receptive to his or her partner's touch. This phenomenon can certainly happen to both partners, but Buehler said it's particularly common for women to report feeling "touched out" after caring for a newborn.

The Baby Came Out Already, Why Does My Pelvis Still Hurt?

Ideally, once your little one has made his or her grand entrance, your pelvic pain should go away. But if you are in the 5 percent to 8 percent of women whose pain persists, you may be wondering why you are still waddling around and what you can do about it. According to recent studies, pregnancy-related pelvic pain can remain until two years after giving birth. And in some cases, it can become chronic and never really go away. Pain in the pelvis can also be very vague, which makes it all the more frustrating. Pain can occur in the front of the pelvis, in the back of the pelvis, or both. It can also refer pain to other parts of your hips and abdomen. There are many reasons this can occur. Everyone has a different pregnancy experience. Some women experience this pain while others don't.

So if you are the unlucky one, what can you do about it? Let's get you out of that 5 percent to 8 percent! There are some "band-aids" that you can use to help ease your discomfort.

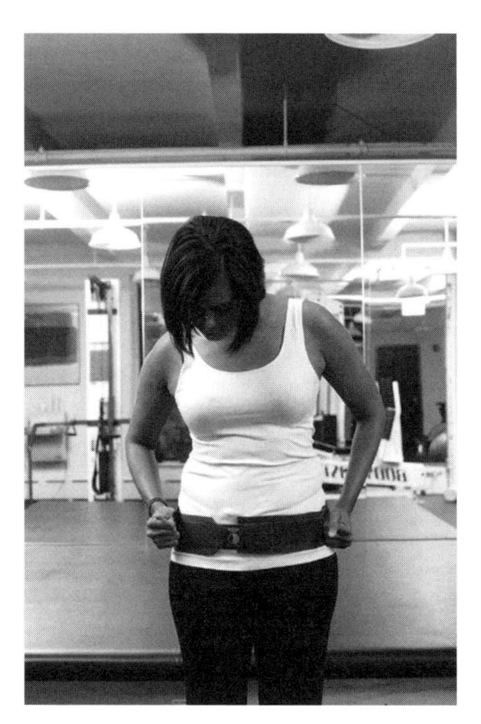

Applying pelvic belt for pelvic pain

- **Pelvic belts** can relieve the stress on ligaments and cartilage in your pelvis by adding compression externally. The belts you choose should have soft material and should fasten with Velcro. We're not talking about the weight lifting belts from your local meathead gym.

One option is the Serola Sacroiliac Belt. This belt has two extra Velcro straps fastened to the midline of the belt. You can pull the ends of the belt tighter in the front *or* flip the belt around and pull the ends tighter in the back. You decide where you need the extra stabilization.

Another option is a pelvic compression belt such as the Com-Pressor Belt developed by Diane Lee that has four separate Velcro straps. The straps are not fastened to the belt. This allows you to apply compression wherever you need it.

Remember to always wear your support belts *over* your clothing. Otherwise, the belt may slide against your skin and cause skin irritation. We don't want to add chafing to your long list of things to worry about!

Conclusion

Look how far you have come. You were swollen like a sausage. Waddling like a duck. Stuck in a chair. Wondering if you were going to make it through the next few months. And you did! And one benefit to pregnancy brain and momnesia is that you can't remember feeling so lousy! Here you are, triumphantly caring for yourself and your new baby(ies). You feel well. You managed your discomforts. You prevented hints of pain from getting worse. You helped your body recover and get stronger. You mended your scars, fixed that residual back pain, and took wonderful care of your little one(s) with perfect technique.

We understand that all this can be very overwhelming. Trying to juggle your newborn(s), home, family, career, and yourself is a tough task to say the least. Taking advice from a few experts on pregnancy is the easy part. How you use the advice is up to you. Do what works best for you. If you can't sneak out to see a women's health physical therapist, acupuncturist, massage therapist, or other specialist, you have some helpful tips that you can do on your own to ease your discomforts. Most importantly, enjoy this special time. Let us be the first of many to tell you, it goes by very quickly.

You are also going to be very prepared for your next pregnancy, which we guess is the last thing on your mind right now. However, when and if that time comes around, you are going to be ready and armed with an arsenal of exercises and solutions to make your next pregnancy, your best pregnancy.

Love,
Denise and Jill

Notes

Chapter 1

Lower Back Pain

p. 9: *According to a recent study: Massage therapy …* Field T. (2010) Pregnancy and labor massage. *Expert Rev Obstet Gynecol* 5(2): 177–181.

Upper Back and Shoulder Pain

p. 10: *Additionally, supportive bras …* Luciani J, Deal A. (2009) *The Bra Book: The Fashion Formula to Finding the Perfect Bra*. Dallas: BenBella Books.

p. 11: *A bra fits well if …* www.BreastCancerCare.org

p. 11: *These types of bras can also be worn …* www.BreastCancerCare.org

p. 11: *According to Jené Luciani …* Luciani J, Deal A. (2009) *The Bra Book: The Fashion Formula to Finding the Perfect Bra.* Dallas: BenBella Books.

Bladder Issues

p. 23: *Reduce or eliminate the urge to urinate …* www.UrologyHealth.org

Carpal Tunnel Syndrome

p. 25: *It was concluded that …* Peterson C, Wacker CA, Phelan T, Blume MK, Tucker R. (2013) Anatomical differences in the shape of the male and female carpal tunnels. *Journal of Women's Health Physical Therapy* 37(3):108–112.

Constipation

p. 29: *Constipation during pregnancy …* Trottier M, Erebara A, Bozzo P. (2012) Treating constipation during pregnancy. *Can Fam Physician* 58(8):836–838.

p. 31: *Pregnant women should drink as much as …* Evan J, Aronson R. (2005) *The Whole Pregnancy Handbook: An Obstetrician's Guide to Integrating Conventional and Alternative Medicine Before, During, and After Pregnancy.* New York City: Gotham Publishing.

p. 31: *The squatting position …* Sikirov D. (2003) Comparison of straining during defecation in 3 positions: Results and implications for human health. *Dig Dis Sci* 48(7):1201–1205.

Heel and Bottom of Foot Pain (Plantar Fasciitis)

pp. 32–33: *It was concluded that pregnancy …* Segal NA, Boyer ER, Teran-Yengle P, et al. (2013) Pregnancy leads to lasting changes in foot structure. *Am J Phys Med Rehabil* 92(3):232–240.

Night Cramps

p. 39: *Studies show that during pregnancy, up to 30 percent …* Hensley JG. (2009) Leg cramps and restless legs syndrome during pregnancy. *J Midwifery Womens Health* 54(3):211–218.

p. 42: *Eighty-six pregnant women participated in a 2012 study …* Supakatisant C, Phupong V. (2012) Oral magnesium for relief in pregnancy-induced leg cramps: A randomised controlled trial. *Maternal & Child Nutrition.*

p. 42: *Another study showed leg cramps …* Sohrabvand F, Karimi M. (2009) Frequency and predisposing factors in pregnancy leg cramps: A prospective clinical trial. *Tehran University Medical Journal* 67(9):661–664.

p. 42: *It was concluded that magnesium levels …* Nygaard IH. (2008) Does oral magnesium substitution relieve pregnancy-induced leg cramps? *Eur J Obstet Gynecol Reprod Biol* 141(1):23–26.

p. 42: *Options that have not been proven …* Young G. (2009) Leg cramps. *Clin Evid (Online)*: 1113.

Pelvic Pain

p. 43: *When people have tightened muscles …* Lucas KR, Polus BI, Rich PS. (2004) Latent myofascial trigger points: Their effect on muscle activation and movement efficiency. *J Bodyw Mov Ther* 8:160–166.

p. 43: Among all the relevant studies ... Kanakaris, M, Giannoudis, PV, Roberts, C. Pregnancy-related pelvic girdle pain: an update. BMC. 2011:9:15.

Pubic Symphysis Pain/Symphysis Pubis Dysfunction (SPD)

p. 47: *However, if the separation is between* … Parker JM, Bhattacharjee M. (2009) Peripartum diastasis of the symphysis pubis. *N Engl J Med* 361:1886.

p. 53: More Pubic Symphysis Relief ... www.pelvicjointpain.org.nz

Separated Abdominal Muscles (Diastasis Recti)

p. 66: *Healthy connective tissue* … Irion JM, Iron G. (2009) *Women's Health in Physical Therapy*. NewYork: Lippincott Williams & Wilkins.

p. 66: *Much of the research on diastases* … Boissonnault JS, Blaschak MJ. (1988) Incidence of diastasis recti abdominis during the childbearing year. *Physical Therapy* 68(7):1082–1086.

p. 67: *Their weakened core can contribute* … Keeler J, Albrect M, Eberhardt L, Horn L, Donnelly C, Lowe D. (2012) Diastasis recti abdominis: A survey of women's health specialists for current physical therapy clinical practice for postpartum women. *JOWHPT* (36):131–142.

Shortness of Breath

p. 76: *Feeling short of breath* … Pereira A, Krieger BP. (2004) Pulmonary complications of pregnancy. *Clin Chest Med*. Jun 25(2):299–310.

Sleeping Pains

p. 82: *These conditions affect* … Beckmann CRB, Herbert W, Laube D, Ling F, Smith R. (2013) *Obstetrics and Gynecology.* New York: Lippincott Williams & Wilkins.

p. 82: *The majority of the pregnant group* … Mills GH, Chaffe AG. (1994) Sleeping positions adopted by pregnant women of more than 30 weeks gestation. *Anesthesia* 49(3):249–250.

p. 83: *According to a study* … Bozzo P, Einarson A, Law R, Maltepe C. (2010) Treatment of heartburn and acid reflux associated with nausea and vomiting during pregnancy. *Canadian Family Physician* 56(2):143–144.

p. 83: *Additionally: Eat slowly* … www.WomensHealth.gov

Swelling

p. 84: *You are carrying around …* Davison JM. (1997) Edema in pregnancy. *Kidney International Supplements* 59:S90– S96.

p. 84: *It is believed there is a shared biologic mechanism …* Costigan KA, Sipsma HL, DiPietro JA. (2006) Pregnancy folklore revisited: The case of heartburn and hair. *Birth* 33(4):311–314.

p. 86: *However, it is not usually as severe …* Sibai BM. (2012) Hypertension. In: Gabbe SG, Niebyl JR, Simpson JL, et al., eds., *Obstetrics: Normal and Problem Pregnancies*. 6th ed. Philadelphia, PA: Saunders Elsevier.

p. 87: *It was concluded that both excessively high …* Koleganova N, Piecha G, Ritz E, et al. (2011, August) Both high and low maternal salt intake in pregnancy alter kidney development in the offspring. *American Journal of Physiology. Renal Physiology* 301(2):F344–354.

Varicose Veins

p. 90: *Varicose veins are a common condition …* Perrot-Applanat M, et al. (1995) Progesterone receptor expression in human saphenous veins. *Circulation* 92:2975–2983.

p. 91: *It was concluded that women with varicose veins …* Lenkovic M, et al. (2009) Effect of progesterone and pregnancy on the development of varicose veins. *Acta Dermatovenerologica Croatica: ADC* 17(4):263–267.

p. 91: *Research, however, shows that women …* Furuta N, Kondoah E, Yamada S, Kawasaki K, Ueda A, Mogami H, et al. (2013) Vaginal delivery in the presence of huge vulvar varicosities: A case report with MRI evaluation. *European Journal of Obstetrics, Gynecology, and Reproductive Biology* 167(2):127–131.

p. 92: *Though they have not been proven to prevent …* Thaler E, Huch R, Huch A, Zimmermann R. (2001) Compression stockings prophylaxis of emergent varicose veins in pregnancy: A prospective randomised controlled study. *Swiss Medical Weekly* 131:659–662.

Chapter 2

p. 101: *In a study of almost 1,500 U.S. women …* Evenson KR, Marshal SW, Vladutiu CJ. (2010, November) Physical activity and injuries during pregnancy. *J Phys Act Health* 7(6):761–769.

p. 103: *Women who engaged in light physical activity …* Hegaard HK, Hedegaard M, Damm P, Ottesen B, Petersson K, Henriksen TB.

(2008) Leisure time physical activity is associated with a reduced risk of preterm delivery. *Am J Obstet Gynecol* 198(2):180 e1–180 e5.

p. 108: *By the end of pregnancy ...* Bloom S, Cunningham F, Leveno K, Hauth J, Rouse D, Spong C. (2009) *Williams Obstetrics*. McGraw Hill: New York.

p. 108: *Nerve fibers that run next to the ligaments ...* Jordan RG, Engestrom J, Marfell J, Farley CL. (2014) *Prenatal and Postnatal Care*. New Jersey: Wiley-Blackwell.

p. 109: *The "talk-test" ...* Clapp JF. (2012) *Exercising Through Your Pregnancy*. Nebraska: Addicus Books.

p. 110: *There is no retrospective evidence ...* Kramer MS. (2006) Aerobic exercise for women during pregnancy. *Cochrane Database Syst Rev* (3):CD000180.

p. 111: *Besides the psychological health benefits ...* American College of Obstetricians and Gynecologists. (2002) Exercise during pregnancy and the postpartum period. American College of Obstetricians and Gynecologists Committee Opinion No. 267. *Obstet Gynecol* 99:171–173.

p. 111: *Some studies show lowered rates ...* Field T, Diego M, Medina L, Delgado J, Hernandez A. (2012) Yoga and massage therapy reduce prenatal depression and prematurity. *Bodyw Mov Ther* 16(2): 204–209.

p. 114: *Strenuous activity can cause torsion ...* Littman ED, Rydfors J, Milki AA. (2003) Exercise-induced ovarian torsion in the cycle following gonadotrophin therapy: Case report. *Hum Reprod* 18 (8):1641–1642.

p. 114: *Research suggests not lifting ...* Hakakha M, Brown A. (2010) *Expecting 411*. Boulder: Windsor Peak Press.

p. 115: *According to the Cleveland Clinic ...* http://my.clevelandclinic.org/healthy_living/pregnancy/hic_correct_posture_and_body_mechanics_during_pregnancy.aspx

p. 116: *If you are unable to speak ...* American College of Sports Medicine. (2013) *ACSM's Resource Manual for Guidelines for Exercise Testing and Prescription*. New York: Lippincott Williams & Wilkins.

p. 117: *It is recommended that pregnant women drink ...* Ehrman J, Gordon P, Visich P, Keteyian S. (2013) *Clinical Exercise Physiology*. Champaign: Human Kinetics.

Chapter 3

p. 120: *The goal is to keep the pelvic floor …* Norton P. (1993) Pelvic floor disorders: The role of fascia and ligaments. *Clin Obstet and Gynecol* 36(4):926–938.

p. 121: *Not only does a strong pelvic floor increase …* Cooper A. (2009) *The Everything Orgasm Book: The All-You-Need Guide to the Most Satisfying Sex You'll Ever Have (Everything Series).* New York City: Adams Media.

Chapter 4

p. 130: *You will also be experiencing a large increase …* Berghella V. (2007) *Obstetric Evidence Based Guidelines.* London: Taylor & Francis Group.

p. 133: *Semen contains prostaglandins …* Kropp T. (2008) *The Joy of Pregnancy: The Complete, Candid, and Reassuring Companion for Parents-to-Be*: Boston: Harvard Common Press.

Chapter 5

p. 137: *Bed rest is one of the most widely used …* Biggio Jr, JR. (2013) Bed rest in pregnancy: Time to put the issue to rest. *Obstet & Gynecol* 121(6):1158–1160.

p. 137: *Approximately 18 percent of pregnant women …* Sciscione AC. (2010) Maternal activity restriction and the prevention of preterm birth. *Am J Obstet Gynecol* 202:232.e1–e5.

p. 142: *This was studied in 713 women …* Crowther CA, Han S. (2010) Hospitalisation and bed rest for multiple pregnancy. *Cochrane Database Syst Rev* Jul 7:(7).

p. 142: *Cochrane reviews of bed rest …* Sosa C, Althabe F, Belizán J, Bergel E. (2004) Bed rest in singleton pregnancies for preventing preterm birth. *Cochrane Database Syst Rev* (1).

p. 142: *The depression lessens …* Maloni JA. (2011, July 1) Lack of evidence for prescription of antepartum bed rest. *Expert Rev Obstet Gynecol* 6(4):385–393.

p. 143: *At least 14.5 percent of women …* Gaynes et al. (2005) Perinatal depression: Prevalence, screening accuracy, and screening outcomes. *Evid Rep/Technol Assess* No. 119 (Summ):1–8.

p. 143: *In addition to these …* American Psychiatric Association. (2013) *Diagnostic and Statistical Manual of Mental Disorders. 5th ed.* Arlington, VA: American Psychiatric Publishing.

p. 143: *Edinburgh Postnatal Depression Scale.* Cox JL, Holden JM, Sagovsky R. (1987) Detection of postnatal depression: Development of the 10-item Edinburgh Postnatal Depression Scale. *Br J Psychiatry* 150:782–786.

p. 145: *Perinatal depression has been associated …* Grigoriadis S, VonderPorten EH, Mamisashvili L, et al. (2013) The impact of maternal depression during pregnancy on perinatal outcomes: A systematic review and meta-analysis. *J Clin Psychiatry* 74(4):e321–e341.

p. 146: *Perinatal depression has been associated …* Grote NK, Bridge JA, Gavin A, et al. (2010) A meta-analysis of depression during pregnancy and the risk of preterm birth, low birth weight, and intrauterine growth restriction. *Arch Gen Psychiatry* 67(10): 1012–1024.

p. 146: *In 2009, after a thorough review …* Yonkers KA, Wisner KL, Stewart DE, et al. (2009) The management of depression during pregnancy: A report from the American Psychiatric Association and The American College of Obstetricians and Gynecologists. *Obstetrics & Gynecology* 114(3):703–713.

p. 146: *In individual studies that have noted …* Grigoriadis S, BonderPorten EH, Mamisashvili L, et al. (2013) Antidepressant exposure during pregnancy and congenital malformations: Is there an association? A systematic review and meta-analysis of the best evidence. *J Clin Psychiatry* 2013;74(4):e293–308.

p. 146: … *review of the literature regarding antidepressant use* … Byatt N, Deligiannidis KM, Freeman MP. (2013) Antidepressant use in pregnancy: A critical review focused on risks and controversies. *Acta Psychiat Scand* 127:94–114.

p. 146: *Studies have shown that severe stress …* Talge NM, Neal C, Glover V, et al. (2007) Antenatal maternal stress and long-term effects on child neurodevelopment: How and why? *J Child Psych Psychiatry* 48:245–261.

Chapter 6

p. 162: *Episiotomies have been linked …* Aukee P, Sundstrom H, Kairalouma MV. (2006) The role of mediolateral episiotomy during labour: Analysis of risk factors for obstetric anal sphincter tears. *Acta Obstet Gynecol Scand* 85(7):856–860.

pp. 162–63: These lacerations can occur … Andrews V, Sultan AH, Thakar R, Jones PW (2006) Occult anal sphincter injuries–myth or reality? *BJOG: An International Journal of Obstetrics and Gynaecology* 113(2): 195–200.

p. 163: *With episiotomies, there is more bleeding …* Eason E, Feldman P. (2000) Much ado about a little cut: Is episiotomy worthwhile? *Obstet Gynecol* 95(4):616–618.

p. 163: *With episiotomies, there is more … scarring …* Koger K, Shatney C, Hodge K, McLenathan J. (1993). Surgical scar endometrioma. *Surgery, Gynecology and Obstetrics* 177(3):243–246.

p. 163: *With episiotomies, there is … increased pain …* Macarthur AJ, Macarthur C. (2004) Incidence, severity, and determinants of perineal pain after vaginal delivery: A prospective cohort study. *Am J Obstet Gynecol* 191(4):1199–1204.

p. 163: *An episiotomy can also be beneficial …* Röckner G, Fianu-Jonasson A. (1999) Changed pattern in the use of episiotomy in Sweden. *Br J Obstet Gynaecol* 106:95.

p. 163: *The rate of episiotomy …* Frankman EA, Wang L, Bunker CH, Lowder JL. (2009) Episiotomy in the United States: Has anything changed? *Am J Obstet Gynecol* 200:573.e1.

p. 163: *It is highest in Latin America …* Carroli G, Belizan J. (2003) Episiotomy for vaginal birth. *Cochrane Database Syst Rev* (3).

p. 163: "*What nature separates …* Sears M, Sears W. (2013) *The Healthy Pregnancy Book: Month by Month, Everything You Need to Know From America's Baby Experts.* New York: Little, Brown & Company.

p. 163: *Antenatal perineal massage reduces …* Beckmann MM, Garrett AJ. (2006, January 25) Antenatal perineal massage for reducing perineal trauma. *Cochrane Database Syst Rev* (1).

p. 163: *One study from 2012 found …* Aasheim V, Nilsen A, Lukasse M, Reinar LM. (2012) Perineal techniques during the second stage of labour for reducing perineal trauma. *Cochrane Summaries.*

p. 165: *Pushing in an upright position …* Gupta JK, Hofmeyr GJ, Shehmar M. (2012, May 16) Position in the second stage of labour for women without epidural anaesthesia. *Cochrane Database Syst Rev* (5).

p. 165: *Even though there are great benefits …* Declercq ER, Sakala C, Corry MP, Applebaum S. (2006) Listening to mothers II: Report of the Second National U.S. Survey of Women's Childbearing Experiences. *J Perinat Educ* 16(4):9–14.

p. 174: *Researchers reviewed the findings …* Souza JP, Miquelutti MA, Cecatti JG, Makuch M. (2006) Maternal position during the first stage of labor: A systematic review. *Reproductive Health* 3:10.

p. 174: … *walking extra-long distances* … Riley L. (2012). *You and Your Baby Pregnancy: The Ultimate Week-by-Week Pregnancy Guide (You & Your Baby)*. Wiley: New Jersey.

p. 174: *It may be due to the physical stimulation* … Rakel D. (2012) *Integrative Medicine*. Saunders: Philadelphia.

Chapter 8

p. 194: symptoms of the "baby blues" … www.Parent2Parent.ca

p. 201: *Studies show that 53 percent of women* … Boissonnault JS, Blaschak MJ. (1988) Incidence of diastasis recti abdominis during the childbearing year. *Physical Therapy* 7(68):1082– 1086.

p. 203: *A substantial number of these women* … Goldstein A, Pukall C, Goldstein I. (2009) *Female Sexual Pain Disorders: Evaluation and Management*. Boston: Wiley-Blackwell.

p. 204: *Dr. Streicher, a leading women's sexual health expert* … Streicher L. (2014) *Love Sex Again A Gynecologist Finally Fixes the Issues That Are Sabotaging Your Sex Life*. New York: It Books.

p. 204: *Out of the 4 million women* … Signorello LB, Harlow BL, Chekos AK, et al. (2001) Postpartum sexual functioning and its relationship to perineal trauma: A retrospective cohort study of primiparous women. *Am J Obstet Gynecol* 184:881–890.

p. 205: *According to a 2013 study* … Fehniger JE, Brown JS, Creasman JM, Feden VD, Stephen K, Thom DH, Subak, L, Huang A. (2013) Childbirth and female sexual function later in life. *Obstetrics & Gynecology* 122(5):988–997.

p. 205: *According to recent studies, pregnancy related pelvic pain* … Kanakaris M, Giannoudis PV, Roberts C. (2011) Pregnancy-related pelvic girdle pain: An update. *BMC* 9:15.

Acknowledgments

We have so many people to thank. Our book wouldn't have been possible without our agent and editor. Thank you, Janet Rosen, for believing in our book and finding us a publisher. Thank you, Julia Pastore, for your keen eye, attention to detail, and tremendous help in polishing our book.

Thank you to our patients for sharing your stories and trusting us with your care. We promise all your names have been changed!

Thank you to Aiden Hoefs, Michael Hoefs, Zoe Hoefs, Sullivan Isola, Lovelyn Palm, Robin Roberts, and Lori Shaw for allowing us to feature you and use your pictures.

Thank you, Bryan Derballa, for our great photographs. You were so patient and helpful when we had "just one more picture" to take. You are fantastic.

Thank you Jill Blakeway, MS, LAc; Sabrina Khan, MD; Nicole Kruck, LMT; Mary Sabo, LAc; Allyson Augusta Shrikhande, MD; and Julie Tupler, RN, for your expert contributions.

Thank you to Sidelines National High Risk Pregnancy Support Network and *Journal of Midwifery & Women's Health* for allowing us to use your valuable patient materials.

Thank you to Graco Children's Products, Inc; It's You Babe, LLC; Kinetic Diversified Industries, Inc; Sakura Bloom, LLC; Squatty Potty, LLC; Medi-Dyne Healthcare Products; Serola Biomechanics, Inc, Ltd; Table for Two, LLC; Tupler, Inc; and Twin Z Company for allowing us to use your products in our book.

And last but certainly not least, thank you to our amazing families.

Jane and Howard Butensky—you were so supportive when I needed to write. Thanks for the love (and babysitting, cooked meals, use of your house ...).

Mr. and Mrs. Jagroo, Sarah, Sagi, Nate and Jess—Thank you for your constant love and support.

Index

About the Authors

Jill Hoefs, MPT, is a physical therapist and owner of Body Align Physical Therapy in both New York City and Summit, New Jersey. Upon graduating from the University of Wisconsin-Madison with a master's degree in physical therapy, Hoefs moved to Manhattan to begin her career. Hoefs loves treating her pregnant patients and helps them during every phase of their pregnancy. She treats their prenatal symptoms, prepares them for labor, and helps their postpartum recoveries. In addition to treating patients, Hoefs teaches classes on childbirth preparation and postpartum recovery. She is a licensed Tupler Technique® provider and specializes in treating diastasis recti. Hoefs lives with her husband and their two children in Summit, New Jersey. She can be reached at jill@bodyalignpt.com.

www.bodyalignpt.com

Denise Jagroo earned her doctoral degree in physical therapy from New York University. She also has a manual therapy certification (MTC) through the University of St. Augustine, a certificate of achievement in pelvic physical therapy, and her board certification as a clinical specialist in Women's Health Physical Therapy (WCS) through the American Physical Therapy Association's Women's Health Section. She lectures nationally to clinicians regarding women's health topics and has been a featured speaker at several national annual physical therapy conferences. She teaches her own course on pelvic health and rehabilitation and workshops on pregnancy, postpartum, and pelvic health topics. Jagroo treats pelvic, obstetric, and orthopedic dysfunctions at her practice in New York City, which includes physical therapy home and office visits. Jagroo is a survivor of pelvic pain. She is now pain free and wrote this book to help women everywhere learn to relieve their own discomforts.

drjagroo.com